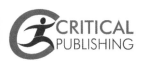

CRITICAL
PUBLISHING

Critical Thinking Skills for your

Nursing Degree

**CRITICAL
STUDY SKILLS**

JANE BOTTOMLEY AND STEVEN PRYJMACHUK

First published in 2018 by Critical Publishing Ltd

British Library Cataloguing in Publication Data
A CIP record for this book is available from the British Library

ISBN: 978-1-912096-69-5

This book is also available in the following e-book formats:

MOBI: 978-1-912096-68-8
EPUB: 978-1-912096-67-1
Adobe e-book reader: 978-1-912096-66-4

Text and cover design by Out of House Limited
Project Management by Out of House Publishing Solutions
Printed and bound in Great Britain by Bell & Bain, Glasgow

Critical Publishing
3 Connaught Road
St Albans
AL3 5RX

www.criticalpublishing.com

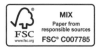

MIX
Paper from
responsible sources
FSC® C007785

Contents

Acknowledgements

We would like to thank the many university and nursing students who have inspired us to write these books. Special thanks are due to Anita Gill. Our appreciation also goes to Lois Gale and her very critical (in a good sense!) nursing postgraduates at the University of Manchester for their invaluable comments, and to Julia Morris at Critical Publishing for her support and editorial expertise.

Jane Bottomley and Steven Pryjmachuk

Meet the authors

Jane Bottomley

is a Senior Language Tutor at the
University of Manchester and a Senior
Fellow of the British Association of
Lecturers in English for Academic
Purposes (BALEAP). She has helped
students from a wide range of disciplines
to improve their academic skills and
achieve their study goals. She has
previously published on scientific writing.

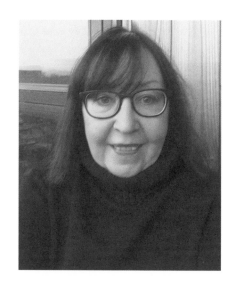

Steven Pryjmachuk

is Professor of Mental Health Nursing
Education in the School of Health
Sciences' Division of Nursing, Midwifery
and Social Work at the University of
Manchester and a Senior Fellow of the
Higher Education Academy. His teaching,
clinical and research work has centred
largely on supporting and facilitating
individuals – be they students, patients
or colleagues – to develop, learn or care
independently.

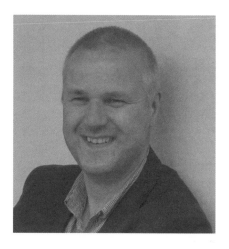

Introduction

Critical Thinking Skills is the third book in the *Critical Study Skills for Nurses* series. This series supports student nurses, midwives and health professionals as they embark on their undergraduate degree programme. It is aimed at all student nurses, including those who have come to university straight from A levels, and those who have travelled a different route, perhaps returning to education after working and/or raising a family. The books will be of use both to students from the UK and to international students who are preparing to study in a new culture – and perhaps in a second language. The books also include guidance for students with specific learning requirements.

Critical Thinking Skills aims to remove some of the 'mystique' which often surrounds critical thinking – students sometimes hear that they are 'not critical' enough but may struggle to understand just what this means in practical terms. This book guides you towards an understanding of critical thinking and its role in academic and professional life, with plain-English explanations and practical examples provided throughout. It discusses the importance of questioning what you see and hear, and equips you with a range of analytical and evaluative tools. It places reflective practice at the heart of critical thinking and provides language tools which can help you express your reflections more precisely. It provides strategies to help you read and write critically, using the research and writing process to discover and develop your own voice, an essential part of being a critical scholar.

Between them, the authors have many years' experience of both nursing practice and education, and academic study skills. All the information, text extracts and activities in the book have a clear nursing focus and are often directly linked to the **Nursing and Midwifery Council's Code**. There is also reference to relevant institutional bodies, books and journals throughout.

The many activities in the book include **tasks**, **reflections**, **top tips**, and **case studies**. There are also **advanced skills** sections, which highlight particular knowledge and skills that you will need towards the end of your degree programme – or perhaps if you go on to postgraduate study. The activities in the book often require you to work things out and discover things for yourself, a learning technique which is commonly used in universities. For many activities, there is no right or wrong answer – they might simply require you to reflect on your experience or situations you are likely to encounter at university; for tasks which require a particular response, there is an answer key at the back of the book.

These special features throughout the book are clearly signalled by icons to help you recognise them:

 Learning outcomes;

 Quick quiz or example exam questions/assessment tasks;

 Reflection (a reflective task or activity);

 Case studies;

Top tips;

 Checklist;

 Advanced skills information;

 Answer provided at the back of the book.

Students with limited experience of academic life in the UK will find it helpful to work through the book systematically; more experienced students may wish to 'dip in and out' of the book. Whichever approach you adopt, handy **cross references** signalled in the margins will help you quickly find the information that you need to focus on or revisit.

There are two **Appendices** (Academic levels at university; Verb tenses in English) at the back of the book, which you can consult as you work through the text.

We hope that this book will help you to develop as a critical nursing student and practitioner, and to become a confident member of your academic community.

A note on terminology

In the context of this book, the term 'nursing' should be taken to include 'nursing, midwifery and the allied health professions', wherever this is not explicitly stated.

Chapter 1
The foundations of critical thinking

Learning outcomes

After reading this chapter you will:

- understand what is meant by 'critical thinking';

- understand the relevance and importance of critical thinking in the theory and practice of nursing;

- have begun to learn how to apply critical thinking to your studies and to your nursing practice.

CROSS REFERENCE

Chapter 2, Reflective practice

There are many books and courses in schools, colleges and universities entitled 'Critical Thinking' (like this book!), a fact which reflects its importance in education, particularly in universities. However, critical thinking is not a discrete study topic like those in other books and modules you may encounter (for example, 'The human body in childbearing' or 'Supporting end-of-life care'); critical thinking is actually threaded through every aspect of your studies and your practice.

CROSS REFERENCE

Chapter 3, Critical reading

This chapter helps you begin to trace and understand this thread. It explores important aspects of critical thinking in academic study and in nursing practice, in particular, the importance of objectively questioning the information and ideas you encounter. Chapter 2 explores reflective practice, which is closely related to critical thinking and is a key aspect of nursing. Chapters 3 and 4 cover how to *apply* critical thinking skills in your academic reading and writing.

Of course, it is not possible to think critically about a nursing topic if you are not grounded in the *knowledge* of your discipline, and all the guidance and tasks in this book will be rooted in your developing knowledge of nursing theory and practice.

CROSS REFERENCE

Chapter 4, Critical writing

Reflection

1) What do you understand by the term 'critical thinking'?

2) Why do you think critical thinking, as you understand it, is so important across education and professional practice?

3) Which parts of the Nursing and Midwifery Council (NMC) Code (2015) make reference to critical thinking?

4) Have you ever received feedback from a teacher or lecturer which said you had not been critical enough? Did you understand what you had done wrong?

5) Have you felt that something you recently read or heard was lacking in critical thinking? Why?

6) In what ways do you think you can demonstrate criticality in your studies and your nursing practice?

Asking the right questions

A good place to start with critical thinking is with the idea of asking questions in order to get to the truth. This idea can be traced back to the ancient Greek philosopher Socrates, who is said to have laid down the roots of western philosophy by questioning everything around him, and by demonstrating time and again that seemingly knowledgeable people, himself included, often didn't really know what they thought they knew!

> An example [of Socrates's questioning approach] was his conversation with Euthydemus. Socrates asked him whether being deceitful counted as being immoral. Of course it does, Euthydemus replied. He thought that was obvious. But what, Socrates asked, if your friend is feeling very low and might kill himself, and you steal his knife? Isn't that a deceitful act? Of course it is. But isn't it moral rather than immoral to do that? It's a good thing, not a bad one – despite being a deceitful act.
>
> (Warburton, 2012, p 2)

Socrates' thinking may seem like common sense: most of us can think of examples of 'deceit' – the telling of 'white lies', for instance – which are intended to help rather than harm people. But the important point is that Socrates was questioning received wisdom and relying solely on reasoned argument to arrive at the truth. The use of questioning and reasoned argument is central to academic and professional practice. This means, in essence, *not believing things merely because someone important says they are true*, and making sure your own beliefs are constructed around sound reasoning and credible evidence.

Knowledge and understanding in science and healthcare are developing all the time. This inevitably means that sometimes there are instances of received wisdom which turn out to be wrong. This may be because not enough was known about a particular thing at a given time, or it may be that people did not ask enough questions – or at least the *right* questions.

Task

Exploring changes in thinking 1

Look at the case studies below and answer these questions:

1) What was the current knowledge or 'received wisdom' in each case?

2) How was this challenged?

3) What, if anything, do you think should happen now?

Case studies

The Nappy Science Gang

When shopping for washing powder in any UK supermarket, we are faced with the choice of biological or non-biological detergents. Many of us may not be sure of the difference between them, but the information generally available to consumers suggests that biological detergents are more powerful and better at removing dirt and stains because they contain enzymes (substances that speed up chemical reactions, in relation to cleaning in this case). Ideal for very dirty items like nappies, you might think. However, NHS advice, as reported through the *NHS Choices* website, has long been to wash babies' nappies in *non-biological* detergent, which seems to reflect the general belief among the UK population that biological detergents irritate the skin. Nappy manufacturers and other organisations traditionally aligned themselves with NHS advice. However, in 2015, *The Guardian* reported that the *Nappy Science Gang*, a citizens' science project supported by the *Wellcome Trust* and the *Royal Society of Chemistry*, had been questioning the NHS advice on detergent use. This group of parents cited studies which appeared to show that biological detergents were no more likely to cause skin irritation than non-biological detergents, with no connection being found between enzymes and skin complaints. They also pointed to the fact that this 'myth' of enzyme irritation appeared not to exist in other countries, where, in fact, it can be pretty difficult to find non-biological detergents. The *Nappy Science Gang* asked *NHS Choices* to investigate the evidence base for the advice they were issuing on their website. After consulting the literature and experts in the field, the NHS reported that they would be changing the advice given on their website. So, as reported in *The Guardian*, thanks to 'a bunch of volunteer mums who wouldn't stop asking questions' (Collins, 2015), and the readiness of the NHS to listen, advice on the *NHS Choices* website now reads: 'There's no evidence that using washing powders with enzymes (bio powders) or fabric conditioners will irritate your baby's skin.'

Take your medicine?

Most people are used to being told by their GPs to be sure to *finish* a course of antibiotics, even if they start to feel better. Many people are also aware that this is connected to the issue of growing antibiotic resistance. However, in 2017, an article in the renowned *British Medical Journal* argued that there was insufficient evidence to support the idea that stopping antibiotic use early encourages antibiotic resistance, and that, in fact, taking antibiotics for longer than necessary may actually increase the risk of resistance (Llewelyn et al, 2017). So should patients now throw away their antibiotics when they start feeling better? Well no. GPs warn against relying on the evidence from a single study (Mundasad, 2017), and the authors of the study themselves merely call for more research to be done to see if there is scope for cutting antibiotic use in the future (Llewelyn et al, 2017). What's more, in terms of individual health, experts such as Professor Helen Stokes-Lampard, leader of the Royal College of General Practitioners, warn people against trusting their feelings completely: just because symptoms clear up, it doesn't mean the underlying infection has been eradicated (Mundasad, 2017).

The two case studies you have analysed are good examples of how experts question or change their thinking when confronted with new evidence. There are many other areas of healthcare where similar developments have occurred, some of them widely publicised in the media, and some of them leading to significant changes in policy by governments or healthcare organisations. Some of these cases cause great controversy and even end up in court! As a nurse, it is important that you not only follow academic thinking on health issues as reported in textbooks and journals, but that you also keep an eye on how these issues are reported in the media. This may enable you, for example, to put yourself in a patient's shoes and understand how their perception of an issue or treatment may have been influenced. It links to sections 2 and 6 of the NMC Code: 'listen to people and respond to their preferences and concerns'.

Task

Exploring changes in thinking 2

1) How, to your knowledge, has general thinking developed on the following topics over time?

- Vaping
- Handwashing in clinical practice
- Natural remedies
- Drinking coffee
- Child birth practices
- Breast feeding
- Immunisation

2) Can you identify any important academic studies in these areas?

3) How have these topics been reported on in the news media?

4) What, if anything, do you think needs to happen now in each case?

Advanced skills

Hegel's dialectic

A philosophical process called Hegel's dialectic quite nicely describes the advancement of knowledge in an academic environment. (Hegel was a nineteenth-century German philosopher; 'dialectic' is a formal word that essentially means 'discussion'.)

As illustrated in Figure 1.1, the dialectic basically states that for every **thesis** (ie idea) there will be an antithesis or antitheses (alternative idea[s]). Following a period of debate (which can last years, decades or centuries), a **synthesis** (a merging or fusing) of these ideas emerges. However, this new synthesis becomes a thesis in its own right and the process starts all over again!

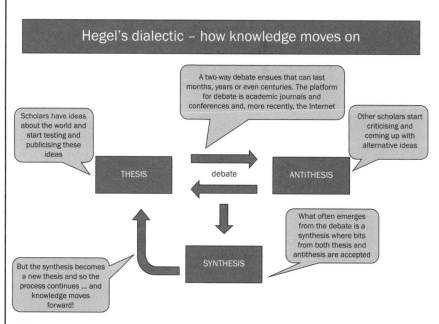

Figure 1.1: Hegel's dialectic

CROSS
REFERENCE

Appendix 1,
Academic
levels at
university

Students at Level 4 (first-year undergraduate students) should be able to demonstrate understanding of one side of the debate. Most students grasp this relatively easily and soon realise that they will get good marks at this academic level if they can convince the person reading (or marking) their work that they understand the concepts, ideas and theories they are writing about.

Level 5 (second-year) students are expected to be aware of the debate between ideas (thesis vs antithesis). Tied in with awareness of this debate is an understanding that there are alternative viewpoints, that there is always another side to the coin, and that if you are going to argue your corner, you must have evidence.

Being able to see how a compromise (synthesis) might be arrived at is a skill that Level 6 (third-year) students need to work towards and it is certainly a skill expected of postgraduate students. This skill is one that few beginners at university have – it's something most acquire as they climb the academic ladder.

At postgraduate level, synthesis is expected to a large extent in that most postgraduate work needs to be underpinned by original thought. This doesn't mean that you spontaneously make up your own theories; it usually means that you've appraised the viewpoints on a specific issue or topic and come up with your ideas about that issue or topic based on what you've read, digested and been convinced by.

Fake news!

The case studies previously discussed in the section on nappies and antibiotics are important in that they show how knowledge and understanding change, and how academics, students and practitioners have a duty to avoid complacency and to keep asking questions. In the case of antibiotics, new evidence has emerged which changes the picture somewhat; in the case of detergents, the evidence was there, but had been overlooked. 'Wrong turns' are part of academic life, and mistakes are made, but in both cases discussed, the parties involved were ostensibly constrained by the rules of academic enquiry, primarily that claims should be *based on evidence*. There was also responsible reporting of the issues in the media outlets concerned. However, this is not always the case! The concept of 'fake news' has come to the fore in recent years. This concept comprises stories that have no basis in fact, but are nevertheless presented as factually accurate – often in order to benefit a particular person or organisation, but sometimes merely to cause mischief and controversy. They can appear in any medium but are particularly common on social media. Fake news stories often focus on politics and celebrity, but they sometimes involve health issues. The influence of this concept was recently highlighted when the *Collins Dictionary* named 'fake news' as the 2017 'word of the year' (Flood, 2017).

Task

Scrutinising the media

Look at the headlines below, taken from news media. Do you know the background behind these headlines? Do you think the stories could be classed as 'fake news'? Why? What questions need to be answered to get to the bottom of the story in each case?

Tumeric helped a dying woman beat cancer

(*Daily Mail*, 24 July 2017)

Drinking three cups of coffee a day can add years to your life

(Metro, 11 July 2017)

Light drinking 'does no harm in pregnancy'

(The Times, 12 September 2017)

Discussion of task

As with most newspaper headlines of this nature, there is actually a grain of truth in the ones cited above. Asking the right questions, however, means doing some detective work to determine if the underlying study or research may have been misinterpreted, or even distorted, by journalists. You might even question whether the journalist or newspaper has a particular political reason (most newspapers have a political stance) or financial reason (controversy breeds publicity!) for running the headline.

One way of probing headlines (or any other statement or claim) is to look for authoritative information on the subject. You might do this by checking out positions from legitimate scientific or professional organisations, or even consulting the original research that led to the headline. Indeed, as you progress through your nursing course, you will find more and more that this is what you are expected to do.

Tumeric helped a dying woman beat cancer

This headline puts two demands on a critically thinking nurse. Firstly, they should be aware of the common bias in human thinking (connected to anecdotal thinking – see case study on page 8: Scientific versus anecdotal thinking) of assuming that an outcome for one specific event will apply more generally. Secondly, evidence from reputable sources should be tracked down. In this case, Cancer Research UK has some useful information that is more balanced: 'There is currently no research evidence to show that turmeric can prevent or treat cancer but early trials have shown some promising results.'

It is notable that Macmillan Cancer Support, the cancer charity, has recently employed a 'digital nurse' to help combat online fake news related to cancer (Silver, 2017).

Drinking three cups of coffee a day can add years to your life

The article relating to this headline refers to an international study looking at half-a-million people across Europe (Gunter et al, 2017). The study concludes that 'coffee drinking was associated with reduced risk for death from various causes' (p 236). The headline is more specific ('three cups'; 'add years to life') than the study conclusion ('associated with reduced risk of death'), but the conclusions are similar. However, a critically thinking nurse would weigh up the pros (very large study, conducted by reputable scientists across many countries) and cons ('risk' and 'associations' are not the same as proof) of this study, and question whether other studies that support or challenge this finding exist before drawing any firm conclusions.

Light drinking 'does no harm in pregnancy'

This headline hit *The Times* newspaper in September 2017, with a report that scientists at the University of Bristol had conducted a study (a systematic literature review) which concluded that there was 'surprisingly limited' proof that a little alcohol harms an unborn baby. The article also quotes David Spiegelhalter, a professor and risk expert at the University of Cambridge, who remarked that any guilt and anxiety felt by women who had an occasional glass of wine should be dispelled by this study.

Broadsheet newspapers like *The Times* tend to have a better reputation for reporting than the tabloid newspapers, but this article created some strong feelings. David Spiegelhalter posted on the social media site Twitter that *The Times* had not included him saying 'precaution is reasonable', which would have markedly changed the tone of the article. Also, the actual conclusions of the University of Bristol study (Mamluk et al, 2017) state that since there is some evidence that light alcohol consumption is associated with smaller babies and premature delivery, abstention as a precautionary principle should remain in any guidance, but that guidance should also say the evidence for the effects of light alcohol consumption is sparse. In other words, *The Times* has confused *no evidence of effect* with *evidence of no effect*. Compare the more inconclusive statement 'the evidence that light alcohol consumption in pregnancy harms unborn babies is limited' with the more definitive statement 'light alcohol consumption does not harm unborn babies'. The headline is thus very misleading. Indeed, the following day, *The Times* published a correction saying the headline had wrongly suggested that light drinking in pregnancy did no harm.

Case study

Scientific versus anecdotal thinking

Shermer (2008) sees the public debate around vaccination and autism as symptomatic of the power of what he calls 'anecdotal thinking', and he suggests quite a compelling reason for this phenomenon:

The recent medical controversy over whether vaccinations cause autism reveals a habit of human cognition – thinking anecdotally comes naturally, whereas thinking scientifically does not. On the one side are scientists who have been unable to find any causal link between the symptoms of autism and the vaccine preservative thimerosal, which in the body breaks down into ethylmercury, the culprit du jour for autism's cause. On the other side are parents who noticed that shortly after having their children vaccinated autistic symptoms began to appear. These anecdotal associations are so powerful that they cause people to ignore contrary evidence: ethylmercury is expelled from the body quickly (unlike its chemical cousin methylmercury) and therefore cannot accumulate in the brain long enough to cause damage. And in any case, autism continues to be diagnosed in children born after thimerosal was removed from most vaccines in 1999; today trace amounts exist in only a few. The reason for this cognitive disconnect is that we have evolved brains that pay attention to anecdotes because false positives (believing there is a connection between A and B when there is not) are usually harmless, whereas false negatives (believing there is no connection between A and B when there is) may take you out of the gene pool.

(Shermer, 2008)

Developing and applying your critical thinking skills

Critical thinking is not peculiar to academia or nursing practice: people are required to use their critical faculties every day in order to make assessments, judgements and decisions. However, in academic and clinical settings, your critical thinking skills will be under particular scrutiny. You will need to consciously develop your critical thinking skills throughout your study and practice, and you will need to draw on these skills in order to complete academic tasks successfully and develop as a nurse. This will involve a range of skills and abilities which you will have to draw on at different stages of your studies and work:

- problem solving, including discussion of ethical issues;

- decision making;

- applying objective criteria to particular situations;

- reflecting on your nursing practice and on your study skills;

- analysing and evaluating sources of information and ideas in terms of suitability, quality and relevance;

- analysing and evaluating information in order to understand a topic;

- identifying, interpreting and assessing the position of other people;

- identifying, interpreting and assessing the arguments put forward by other people to determine if

    - they are well thought through

    - they are reasoned and balanced

    - they are supported with sound, relevant evidence

    - they lead to logical conclusions;

- identifying, interpreting and assessing contrasting points of view;

- evaluating the strength and relevance of the evidence put forward to support different points of view;

- using academic sources to develop your own position (or 'stance') in relation to the topics you will investigate, and presenting (or 'voicing') this stance in a way that will convince a critical reader;

- developing arguments to support your stance which are well thought through, reasoned and balanced;

- finding sound, relevant evidence to support your arguments.

All of the above are explored in later chapters in this book.

CROSS REFERENCE

Chapter 3, Critical reading

CROSS REFERENCE

Chapter 4, Critical writing

Critical thinking in nursing practice

Critical thinking is inherent in the NMC Code (2015) and you should be guided by the Code in your day-to-day practice. You should also bear the Code in mind, and make reference to it, when discussing nursing practice in academic work. The following sections of the Code are particularly explicit as regards the importance of critical thinking.

1.3 Avoid making assumptions and recognise diversity and individual choice.

6.1 Make sure that any information or advice given is evidence based.

8.4 Work with colleagues to evaluate the quality of your work and that of your team.

9.2 Gather and reflect on feedback from a variety of sources, using it to improve practice and performance.

13.1 Accurately assess signs of normal or worsening physical health in the person receiving care.

19.2 Take account of current evidence, knowledge and developments in reducing mistakes and the effect of them.

20.6 Stay objective and have clear professional boundaries at all times with people in your care (including those who have been in your care in the past) and their families and carers.

Task

Applying the NMC Code to critical thinking

1) Compare a nurse saying 'Aromatherapy is great for nausea; I use it myself' with 'We know from some of the research carried out that inhaling ginger or peppermint oil vapour can help with nausea; it seems to work well for a lot of patients though some people don't benefit'. Which statement is more in line with the Code? Why?

2) Many people who have a psychosis (eg schizophrenia) put on weight because a common side-effect of the anti-psychotic medications they take is an increase in appetite. How would you respond if a service user said to their nurse: 'Why should I carry on taking these when they make me fat?'

3) The benefits of 'mindfulness' have been much discussed in the media in recent years. Would you recommend this practice to patients?

Discussion of task

The numbers in brackets are cross references to the sections of the Code mentioned earlier.

1) The second statement is more in line with the Code; the first is a personal anecdote while the second is a more accurate reflection of the evidence base

(6.1). The second statement is better at helping patients make individual choices as to whether to use aromatherapy or not (1.3). Bearing in mind that many patients will see nurses as authoritative, the second statement also doesn't put as much pressure on patients to choose (20.6).

2) Think about the Code when considering the issue.

- Don't assume people will take medication with unpleasant side-effects just because it has been prescribed (1.3; 13.1).

- Weigh the risks of taking the medication against benefits including relief from unpleasant symptoms such as hallucinations and disordered thought, reduced likelihood of being hospitalised, and increased ability to live independently (6.1; 19.2; 20.6).

- Explore ways of helping the service user lose weight (eg through diet and exercise) while they continue to take the medication. Make sure that your suggestions are evidence based (6.1), that they take account of individual needs and preferences (1.3), and that the situation is adequately monitored to track the effects of any actions (13.1).

3) 'Mindfulness' can mean many things, from a formal, evidence-based intervention like Mindfulness-Based Stress Reduction or Mindfulness-Based Cognitive Behaviour Therapy, to informal, often commercial, Buddhist-inspired short courses on meditation or simple one-off activities. The evidence for mindfulness is mixed and, while it may work for some individuals, it may not work for others. It is also not without risks (Shonin et al, 2014). Your recommendation would need to incorporate all of these observations, ie mindfulness can mean many things, the evidence is mixed, some people will benefit from it but others may be harmed by it. An example recommendation, compatible with the Code, would be something like:

> Mindfulness seems to work for some people but not everyone and in some cases it can make things worse for some people (6.1). It might be worth trying it but you should check out the credibility of the course or activity by looking for official (eg NHS, NICE or GP) endorsement rather than, say, celebrity endorsement. If you do decide to enrol on a mindfulness course and you don't seem to be getting any benefit or, indeed, start to feel worse, then stop the course and seek advice from your GP or other healthcare professional (13.1; 19.2).

Reflection

1) Try to think of more incidences where the aspects of the NMC Code discussed in the previous section would be applicable.

2) Think of any practical steps you could take to ensure you follow the guidelines.

3) What **questions** might you want to ask (and to whom) to help you take the best course of action?

Applying critical thinking to ethical issues

As a nurse, you will encounter many difficult or emotive situations and it is important that you respond in a balanced fashion, ie that you manage to be both compassionate and objective. You will be expected to approach these situations critically, to question when necessary, to analyse and evaluate the situation, and to provide reasoned argument to support the position you adopt. It is also necessary to listen to the arguments of others involved in the situation, and to appraise them critically.

Task

Critically appraising ethical concerns

Look at case study A below, based on a real-world referral to the NMC, and answer the questions which follow.

Case study A

'A', a person diagnosed with a borderline personality disorder, was on an acute mental health ward on which 'Z', a mental health nurse, worked. On a night shift, A approached Z and stated that she wanted to self-harm.

After a discussion with A, Nurse Z provided A with a razor blade with which to self-harm. Nurse Z later reported this incident during the handover to the morning staff at the end of her shift. The incident contravened what was in A's care plan (which focused mainly on a therapy called 'dialectical behaviour therapy' or 'DBT').

Nurse Z did not check the wound after A had self-harmed.

Nurse Z made the decision to allow A to self-harm in a supposedly safe way. Do you think Nurse Z's decision was underpinned by critical thinking?

Discussion of case study A

This case went to an NMC Fitness to Practise panel a few years ago and concerns a controversial treatment in mental health called 'harm minimisation'. The theory is that people who self-harm will do so anyway, so it is best to ensure that, when they do it, they do it as safely as possible, ie that they are provided with a clean blade and sterile dressings to clean up afterwards.

The NMC decided to record a caution against the nurse for 12 months, not because the nurse assisted in harm minimisation (though controversial, there is some evidence for it) but because they had contravened the service user's care plan. So while Nurse Z might have used the evidence on harm minimisation to support their decision (6.1), Nurse Z did not take into account competing information (A's care plan) (9.2) or understand the consequences of the decision (A's wounds would need checking) (13.1). This suggests that Nurse Z lacked critical insight when making the decision.

Task

Critically appraising ethical concerns

Look at case study B below, and answer the question that follows.

Case study B

Zara is a 15 year-old secondary school student who confides in Sally, the School Health Adviser (School Nurse) at her school, that she thinks she might be pregnant. She is very upset and asks for advice, at the same time pleading with Sally not to tell her parents, who would, according to Zara, 'go ballistic'.

What information would Sally need to be aware of to help Zara?

Discussion of case study B

Sally would clearly need to know about her obligations according to the Code. In particular, Section 5 is very explicit about confidentiality. Indeed, Sub-section 5.5 gives some additional hints as to what other information Sally would need in order to make informed decisions in relation to Zara:

> 5.5 share with people, their families and their carers, **as far as the law allows**, the information they want or need to know about [emphasis added]

Sally would thus need to know what the law and legal precedents say about the rights of those under 18 (ie those who are legally children) to make their own decisions. Those working with under 18s would certainly need to know about 'Gillick competency' and 'Fraser guidelines', legal precedents that state that children under 18 can be mature enough to make their own health decisions without their parents knowing or being informed. Sally would also probably be aware of the evidence around building trusting relationships with patients and service users, but she would have to balance this against any safeguarding information or obligations, eg protecting Zara from child sexual exploitation.

Reflection

Public investigations into poor practice, such as the Francis Report (2013) on care failings in Mid-Staffordshire, and the Mazars Report (2015) on the failure to investigate unexpected deaths at Southern Health, an NHS mental healthcare provider, have led to a great deal of professional introspection regarding core values. Nurses have a responsibility to view what is going on around them critically so that they can identify poor practice and act accordingly.

What action could you take if you spotted something which concerned you in your placement area or workplace?

Top tips

Exploiting opportunities to hone your critical thinking skills

1) Seminars are an important part of teaching and learning in universities. They are a way of checking your knowledge and understanding, and usually relate directly to lectures and assessments. Importantly, they can provide a space for you to develop your critical thinking skills. They can provide a great opportunity to question others and to test your own ideas in preparation for essays and presentations.

2) Exercise your mind by playing 'devil's advocate'. If your instincts seem to lead you to a particular point of view, try to find arguments and evidence to support the other side. You may not change your mind, but your position will be stronger because you will have tested it.

3) Always try to find the assumptions that lie behind any position. Ask yourself if these assumptions need to be questioned.

4) Don't equate authority or confidence with reason: an authoritative or confident person may be right or wrong. Judge them on the *facts*.

Summary

This chapter has explored the nature of critical thinking in academia and healthcare with reference to real-life case studies. It has focused on the importance of questioning and reasoned argument, and it has introduced strategies for developing and applying critical thinking skills. It has highlighted the centrality of critical thinking in the NMC Code (2015) and in nursing practice. The following chapters further explore these issues.

References

Cancer Research UK (n.d.). Turmeric [online]. Available at: www.cancerresearchuk. org/about-cancer/cancer-in-general/treatment/complementary-alternative-therapies/ individual-therapies/turmeric (accessed 5 March 2018).

Collins, S (2015) The nappy science gang that took on the NHS. *The Guardian*, 30 November [online]. Available at: www.theguardian.com/science/sifting-the-evidence/ 2015/nov/30/nappy-science-gang-versus-the-nhs (accessed 5 March 2018).

Flood, A (2017) Fake news is 'very real' word of the year for 2017. *The Guardian*, 2 November [online]. Available at: www.theguardian.com/books/2017/nov/02/fake-news-is-very-real-word-of-the-year-for-2017 (accessed 5 March 2018).

Francis Report (2013) *Mid-Staffordshire NHS Foundation Trust inquiry*. London: HMSO.

Gunter, M J et al (2017) Coffee drinking and mortality in 10 European countries: a multinational cohort study. *Annals of internal medicine*, 167: 236–47. doi:10.7326/ M16-2945 [online]. Available at: www.ncbi.nlm.nih.gov/pubmed/28693038 (accessed 5 March 2018).

Llewelyn, M, Fitzpatrick, J, Darwin, E, Tonkin-Crine, S, Gorton, C, Paul, J, Peto, T, Yardley, L, Hopkins, S and Walker, A (2017) The antibiotic course has had its day. *BMJ*, 358 [online]. Available at: www.bmj.com/content/358/bmj.j3418 (accessed 5 March 2018).

Mamluk L et al (2017) Low alcohol consumption and pregnancy and childhood outcomes: time to change guidelines indicating apparently 'safe' levels of alcohol during pregnancy? A systematic review and meta-analyses. *BMJ Open*, 7:e015410 [online]. Available at: http://bmjopen.bmj.com/content/bmjopen/7/7/e015410.full.pdf (accessed 5 March 2018).

Mazars (2015) *Independent review of deaths of people with a learning disability or mental health problem in contact with Southern Health NHS Foundation Trust April 2011 to March 2015*. London: Mazars LLP.

Mundasad, S (2017) Should you finish a course of antibiotics? *BBC*, 27 July [online]. Available at: www.bbc.co.uk/news/health-40731465 (accessed 5 March 2018).

Nappy Science Gang (n.d.). A citizen science project about cloth nappies [online]. Available at: https://nappysciencegang.wordpress.com/ (accessed 5 March 2018).

NHS Choices (n.d.) [online]. Available at: www.nhs.uk/pages/home.aspx (accessed 5 March 2018).

Nursing and Midwifery Council (2015) *The Code: professional standards of practice and behaviour for nurses and midwives* [online]. Available at: www.nmc.org.uk/globalassets/sitedocuments/nmc-publications/nmc-code.pdf (accessed 5 March 2018).

Shermer, M (2008) Wheatgrass juice and folk medicine [online]. Available at: https://michaelshermer.com/2008/08/wheatgrass/ (accessed 5 March 2018).

Shonin, E, Van Gordon, W and Griffiths, M (2014) Editorial: are there risks associated with using mindfulness in the treatment of psychopathology? *Clinical Practice*, 11(4), 389–92.

Silver, K (2017) The nurse hired to combat cancer myths online. *BBC*, 30 October [online]. Available at: www.bbc.co.uk/news/health-41780776 (accessed 5 March 2018).

Warburton, N (2012) *A little history of philosophy*. New Haven, CT; London: Yale University Press.

Chapter 2
Reflective practice

Learning outcomes

After reading this chapter you will:

- understand what is meant by the terms 'reflection' and 'reflective practice';

- understand how reflection and reflective practice are an inherent part of critical thinking;

- have gained insight into a number of models of reflective practice and be able to apply them critically;

- be familiar with the characteristics of reflective writing and be able to produce reflective writing which demonstrates these characteristics.

Reflection is the critical analysis of a situation or event, focusing on your own experience, perceptions, behaviour and thought processes. It is a way of making sense of your experience and relating it to your wider studies and professional development.

Practice-based disciplines like nursing have long promoted reflection and regarded it as an important aspect of critical thinking. What's more, reflection is gaining increasing importance across all academic subjects. You will notice that in this book there are a number of 'reflection' tasks which require you to think about your own experiences, abilities and beliefs. These tasks have been included because we, the authors, believe that reflection forms an important part of studying, and of critical thinking in particular. Your assessments at university will almost certainly include reflective essays and shorter accounts which may form part of your professional portfolio or a reflective journal. This chapter will help you to develop your reflective skills and thus enhance both your nursing studies and your nursing practice.

CROSS
REFERENCE

Studying for your Nursing Degree, Chapter 3, Becoming a member of your academic and professional community, The nursing community, Reflective practice

CROSS
REFERENCE

Studying for your Nursing Degree, Chapter 6, Assessment

Reflection and reflective practice

In nursing, you will be expected to reflect on your experience of practice, good and bad, and to write about it. Reflection is slightly unusual among the critical skills you are encouraged to develop at university in that it requires an explicit acknowledgement and analysis of your *emotional* as well as intellectual responses: how you *feel* as well as what you think.

Through reflection, you will be expected to demonstrate a developing understanding of your practice so that you can grow as a practitioner. This may involve better understanding of:

- how to meet the needs of patients;
- what constitutes successful care and how it can be achieved, maintained and replicated;
- how to use resources effectively;
- your own motivation and actions, and the consequences of those actions;
- your own values, beliefs and attitudes;
- how to understand people and their background, and be sensitive to cultural diversity;
- how to work better with patients and their loved ones;
- how to work better with colleagues and partner organisations;
- the origins or root causes of problems;
- decision-making and problem-solving processes.

Reflection

1) What experience do you have so far of reflective activities in your studies or of reflective practice? How did you feel about these experiences?

2) Do you think of yourself as a naturally reflective person, or do you find reflection difficult?

Reflective frameworks

There are a number of reflective models designed to help students think things through in a structured manner. In nursing, there are three which are very widely used:

- **Borton**'s model of structured reflection;
- **Gibbs**' reflective cycle;
- **Johns**' model of structured reflection.

Borton's model of structured reflection

Borton's model of structured reflection is a very simple framework consisting of just three questions:

1) What?
2) So what?
3) Now what?

The 'What?' stage is the description stage, where the situation or event is simply described. The 'So what?' stage is an analytical stage, where you examine why the situation or event was important to you. The 'Now what?' stage is the action stage, where you think about how you might change your practice in the future.

Gibbs' reflective cycle

Gibbs' reflective cycle is a well-known and widely used reflective framework. It was heavily influenced by **Kolb's learning cycle** (Kolb et al, 1991), a way of explaining how people learn through experience. This concept is known as **experiential learning**.

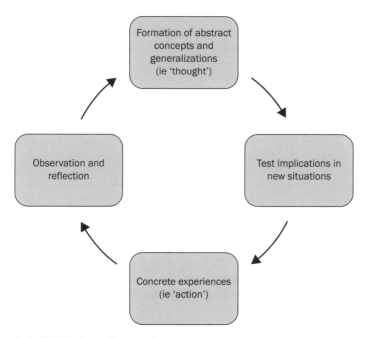

Figure 2.1: Kolb's learning cycle (adapted from Kolb et al, 1991, p 59)

Kolb argues that learning is a **cyclical process** involving a continuous dialogue between thoughts and actions (or theory and practice), mediated by two processes: testing and reflection. In other words, in experiential learning, you test out your ideas in practice, reflect on what goes well and not so well, readjust your ideas if need be, and subsequently test them out. Importantly for practice-based disciplines like nursing, Kolb's model implies that students will struggle to link theory to practice effectively without reflective skills.

Kolb's learning cycle has been highly influential in higher education, and many teachers and students find it very useful. However, like any theory, it must be viewed critically, and, in fact, some scholars have criticised it for being somewhat simplistic, selective and lacking in empirical support. See Tennant (1997) for views on both sides.

Gibbs' model (influenced by Kolb) is also cyclical.

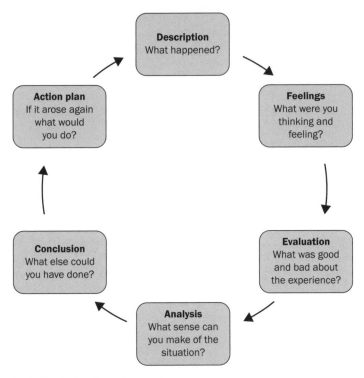

**Figure 2.2: Gibbs' reflective cycle
(adapted from Gibbs, 1988, p 50)**

Gibbs' model has six stages, all of which (except perhaps description) require
a degree of critical thought or analysis about the particular situation you are
interested in. For example, the 'feelings' stage requires you to note how you feel
(angry, upset, overjoyed, anxious, etc) and then think about whether the feelings
were appropriate, or perhaps an under- or over-reaction; the 'analysis' stage
is about you trying to make sense of the situation; and the 'conclusion' stage is
about exploring whether there were alternative ways to deal with the situation.

Johns' model of structured reflection

Christopher Johns, a professor of nursing at the University of Bedfordshire, has
been very influential in the field of reflective practice in healthcare. In contrast
to Gibbs' cyclical approach, Johns' model is linear in nature. It is based upon a
series of questions and cues which practitioners can work through when thinking
about, ie *reflecting on*, a particular situation or event. The questions and cues are
as follows (adapted from Johns, 2009).

- Bring the mind home (a preparatory cue to put you in the best frame of mind to
  reflect).
- Focus on a description of an experience that seems significant in some way.
- Which issues are significant and need attention?
- How do I interpret the way people were feeling and why they felt that way?

- How was I feeling and what made me feel that way?
- What was I trying to achieve and did I respond effectively?
- What were the consequences of my actions on the patients, others and myself?
- What factors influenced the way I was/am feeling, thinking and responding to the situation?
- What knowledge informed me or might have informed me?
- To what extent did I act for the best and in tune with my values?
- How does the situation connect with previous experiences?
- How might I reframe the situation and respond more effectively if a similar situation were to reoccur?
- What would be the consequences of alternative actions for the patients, others and myself?
- What factors might constrain me when responding in new ways?
- How do I NOW feel about this experience?
- Am I more able to support myself and others better as a consequence?
- What insights have I gained?
- Am I more able to realise desirable practice?

Critically evaluating reflective frameworks

The reflective models outlined in the previous section have different approaches, but cover a lot of the same ground. It is useful to analyse the models and compare their approaches and terminology in order to establish which, if any, will work best for you.

Task

Comparing and contrasting reflective frameworks

Look back at the descriptions of the three reflective models outlined in the previous section and, using Borton's simple model as a starting point, complete a table like the one below with comparable elements where possible.

BORTON	GIBBS	JOHNS
What?		
So what?		
Now what?		

Now that you have analysed the three models, you are better placed to evaluate them so that you can decide how useful they will be to you in your study and practice.

Task

CROSS
REFERENCE

*Studying for
your Nursing
Degree,*
Chapter 2,
Strategies
for effective
learning,
Learning
styles

Evaluating reflective frameworks

List the strengths and weaknesses of each model, and relate them to your own learning style or preferences. For example, you might feel that one model provides more or less support than the others, which might be a strength or weakness, depending on how much support you feel is appropriate. Or you may feel that you work better with linear models such as Borton's or Johns', rather than a cyclical model such as Gibbs' – or vice versa: this would be related to your own learning preferences, rather than being a strength or weakness. Use a table like the one below to record your evaluation.

	STRENGTHS	WEAKNESSES	RELATION TO PERSONAL PREFERENCES
Borton			
Gibbs			
Johns			

Reflection *in* action and reflection *on* action

In education circles, Schön's work on reflective practice, *Educating the Reflective Practitioner* (1983), is regarded as a seminal text. Schön distinguishes between reflection *in* action and reflection *on* action. Pryjmachuk (2011, p 67) expands on this in relation to mental health professionals in particular, but this can be applied to all healthcare professionals:

> Reflection on action happens after the event; reflection in action happens during the event. Reflection on action is a prerequisite to becoming a competent practitioner; reflection in action, on the other hand, is a deeper skill that is essential if you are to become a capable practitioner.

Therefore, at the beginning of your studies, you will usually learn to reflect retrospectively *on* action as soon as possible, probably with reference to the models discussed in the previous section. Reflection *in* action, occurring in real time, will be something that you work towards and implement more fully as you progress through your studies, and, indeed, once you practise as a qualified health professional. Both require the critical skills of analysis and evaluation as you strive to make sense of your experience and what is happening around you.

Reflection on learning

It is important that you identify and benefit from the many opportunities at university to reflect on your own learning, and that you use these to improve your knowledge, understanding and performance.

One frequently overlooked opportunity is **feedback** from lecturers or even peers. This could include oral feedback in class or a tutorial, or written feedback on a piece of writing. Writing feedback from a lecturer could be on a first writing draft to help you make improvements before you hand it in, or it could be to explain and justify the mark you were given for an assessment. It is important that you are open to feedback, which will be easier if you manage not to take criticism too personally; it is also important that you take time to analyse and reflect on feedback, and that you use it to develop. Feedback from peers can also be helpful, especially if you are working collaboratively on a group presentation or report; just be careful that collaboration doesn't turn into something which could be interpreted as collusion.

CROSS REFERENCE

Studying for your Nursing Degree, Chapter 6, Assessment, Feedback on academic work

Clinical supervision

One method of enhancing reflective practice that has been especially influential among the healthcare professions is **clinical supervision**. Clinical supervision has its roots in counselling and psychotherapy and is an approach whereby a practitioner meets regularly with a supervisor to discuss and reflect on their caseload or clinical practices. It was very popular in nursing during the 1990s and early 2000s, with the NMC embracing it and arguing that it is an integral part of lifelong learning. As the NMC state (2002, p 7), clinical supervision 'aims to bring practitioners and skilled supervisors together to reflect on practice, to identify solutions to problems, to increase understanding of professional issues and, most importantly, to improve standards of care'. Although clinical supervision is seen as good practice, it is not compulsory in healthcare organisations and it can be quite resource intensive. This means that many employers choose not to incorporate it as a key part of working life, though a fair few employers (the better ones, some would argue) continue to embrace it.

The word 'supervision' can throw up images of surveillance or monitoring, but that is not what clinical supervision aspires to. In fact, it is not about checking what you are doing or identifying poor practice (though it can help you to improve your practice); it is about nurturing you as a healthcare professional and helping you to grow and develop your professional life through experience and reflection.

A clinical supervisor is distinct from a mentor and from a line manager. A mentor is someone who is more experienced than you and who has undergone additional training so that they can support learning and assessment in practice. The fact that they are often involved in assessing you means that they are not in a position to provide clinical supervision in the developmental sense (though their feedback can still help you to develop). A line manager has a formal management role in an organisation, and while a good line manager will encourage and support your professional development, the formal nature of the relationship would not allow them to engage in clinical supervision. Clinical supervision is, in fact, often provided by external agencies such as charities or other NHS trusts, rather than by someone working in the same place as you.

Writing reflectively

As a student nurse, you will be expected to write reflectively in a number of assessments. You may be required to write reflective essays or to provide short reflective accounts, often for your professional portfolio. Some modules may require you to complete a reflective diary, sometimes called a journal or log. Student nurses are often asked to use the reflective models described earlier in this chapter to help them reflect on their experience and organise their ideas in writing.

Short written reflections

CROSS REFERENCE

Academic Writing and Referencing for your Nursing Degree, Chapter 1, Academic writing: text, process and criticality, Writing short reflections for journals and portfolios

In this section, you will analyse short written reflections which would typically appear in a nursing student's professional portfolio or reflective journal.

Task

Identifying appropriate and effective reflections

Compare each pair (A and B) of written reflections below. Which one is more appropriate and effective? Why?

1) **A** Failed my biosciences exam today. Thought I would. Should have studied more and partied less.

   B Failed my biosciences exam today. Thought I would. Can't believe that Sanjita passed it. Grossly unfair.

2) **A** That was really hard; I'm sure everyone thought I was rubbish. I couldn't stop shaking and couldn't look anyone in the face. I'm sure two of my classmates were whispering to each other throughout the presentation. Couldn't wait to get away. Never want to do anything like that again.

   B That was hard. Afterwards, I wondered what my classmates thought about how I did. So I asked them! And I was pleasantly surprised to find that they thought I did well, though one or two said I seemed very nervous. I'm certainly going to ask for feedback when faced with similar situations in the future.

3) **A** Got 85 per cent for my acute care assignment. I knew it was good and I deserved that mark. The marker said that it was an excellent piece of work and that I should be proud of myself. If the marker hadn't given me such a high mark I would have been really upset and angry

as I have put a huge amount of work into this, looking at lots of books and journal articles, and reading the assignment guidelines carefully.

B Got 85 per cent for my acute care assignment. I felt really good about this because I had put a lot of work into it, looked at lots of books and articles, and read the assignment guidelines carefully. The marker said that it was an excellent piece of work and that I should be proud of myself. I am really proud! I'll certainly use the same study strategies for my next piece of work, which will hopefully be as good but, if not, I'll reappraise the situation then.

4) A Today, I received a thank you card from one of the patients I had nursed. It was a really nice card – quite an expensive one with flowers and bows on the front. No-one else on placement with me got one. Went home feeling really good as a result.

B Received a thank you card from one of the patients today. Said I was 'warm, a good listener and caring'. As a student nurse, comments like those mean so much to me as they are the qualities of a good nurse. I was thrilled that a stranger saw them in me.

5) A Met with my academic adviser today. She told me off about my attendance which, admittedly, hasn't been very good recently. We had quite a useful discussion where she explained why attendance was important. I told her that other people skived and didn't seem to get found out. She asked why I was concerned with other people's attendance. I told her that it made me annoyed when other people 'got away with it'. She explained really well why I should focus on me and my behaviour and not worry too much about others. That really made me think. Success on this course depends on me; I must stop making excuses and pull my socks up!

B Met with my academic adviser today. She told me off about my attendance which, admittedly, hasn't been very good recently. Everyone else skives and they don't get found out. Some in my group have missed loads of sessions and nothing seems to happen to them. Feel a bit peeved about this issue. She kept harping on about the 'regulatory body regulations', 'my responsibility' and 'being treated like an adult'. Tried telling me other people's attendance was not really my business. Well I think it is when they get away with it! Might ask for a change of academic adviser if she tries to call me in again.

6) A Attended my first placement (which was with the District Nurses) today. Visited several people in the North Sector and helped change some dressings. Some of the patients – like the lady who had had eight children and the Asian mother whose children had to translate for her – were really interesting. And the way some people live! Absolutely

no furniture in one house! The placement was fab! Would love to be a District Nurse now. It's so interesting and varied. May well choose it for my optional placement in the second year if I'm allowed to.

B Attended my first placement with the District Nurses today. I was quite anxious about it and thought I'd annoyed my mentor by asking loads of questions. We made several home visits and I watched my mentor as she interacted with the patients and undertook her duties. In particular, I was impressed with how the interactions seemed so natural, and, while watching, was trying to work out what it was that the mentor did that made her so effective. Going to talk to her tomorrow to see if she can explain her 'secrets'.

7) A My mentor (a sister on the ward) told me off today about wearing too much jewellery. I explained that I didn't think it was too much. She showed me the Trust's uniform policy and explained about health and safety aspects. I was quite upset (and a bit angry) at first and apologised, but she said I didn't need to apologise, that I was a beginner, that her concerns were only about adhering to the Trust's health and safety policy, and that none of this would affect my assessment in practice. Felt a bit better afterwards and began to understand why she had confronted me.

B Sister dressed me down today for wearing too much jewellery. Called me into the office, sat me down, told me off, showed me the Trust's uniform policy, and explained about health and safety aspects. Suppose she's right but she's one to talk with her nails and rings. She's just got it in for me I know. I really hate this placement. Can't wait to go somewhere less restrictive where the staff are much nicer and are not concerned about picking on people just because they're wearing some jewellery or have the wrong colour shoes or tights.

Discussion of task

1) A is the more reflective response because the student acknowledges that their own behaviour may have had an impact on the outcome and understands that trying to change this behaviour could lead to a different (more positive) outcome.

2) B is the most reflective because there is some attempt to analyse how the experience made the student feel, and the student has demonstrated how their learning might be enhanced by the experience.

3) B is the most reflective because there is some depth of thought given to how the experience made the student feel, and the student has demonstrated how their learning might be enhanced by the experience. A is a little self-centred and superficial.

4) B is a better reflection because the focus is on matching the 'reality' to the expectations of being a nurse. It also shows that the student is receptive to noticing the things that patients value. A is descriptive, and even though the student says they felt good, it's somewhat shallow.

5) A is the most reflective because the student clearly thinks about the situation, listens to other people's points of view, and tries to pull these together to work out how their learning might be enhanced as a consequence. B isn't really reflective because the student can't see the relationship between responsibility and their own learning.

6) B is much more reflective because it is deeper than the mere description that occurs in A. Unlike A, in B, there is focus on the student's feelings and some analysis of how the student's learning might be enhanced.

7) A is the better reflection because feelings are analysed, viewpoints are acknowledged, and the student tries to connect it all to her learning and development. B is judgemental, descriptive and rather petty.

Top tips

Preparing to write reflections

1) Consider the **purpose** of the reflection.

2) Use a **reflective model** or framework (such as Borton's, Gibbs' or Johns') if it helps you organise and deepen your reflection. Adapt the model to suit your own learning preferences.

3) Keep **clear records**, maintaining **anonymity** throughout.

4) Decide the right **time** to write up your reflection – leave enough time for you to have some distance between you and the situation or event, but not so much time that your memory is negatively impacted.

Longer written reflections and essays

In this section, you will analyse a longer written reflection which might typically form part of a reflective essay.

Task

Analysing reflective writing

Read the reflective account below and analyse it with reference to one of the reflective models described earlier in the chapter.

CROSS
REFERENCE

Academic Writing and Referencing for your Nursing Degree, Chapter 1, Academic writing: text, process and criticality, Writing essays, Reflective essays

My last placement was with the school nursing team in [town name not included to maintain anonymity]. I spent most of the time in a mixed ability secondary school, a placement I wasn't really looking forward to as a children's nurse because I prefer working with younger children who have complex physical health problems.

One of the things that struck me immediately about my placement was the number of teenagers with mental health problems. This unnerved me at first as I don't really know enough about mental health problems in children and young people, and I tend to ignore or avoid kids who come into the paediatric wards with these problems because I don't know what to do with them.

One day during my second week of placement, a 14-year-old girl (I'll call her 'Amy', which is not her real name) was brought into the nurse's office with blood all down her arms and over her school shirt. She had been self-harming (cutting herself) and was quite visibly upset. My immediate reaction was to call for an ambulance as I thought this was clearly a medical emergency, but my mentor, Deb (also a pseudonym), said there was no need to call for an ambulance because the cuts were superficial and Amy had cut before. This made me uncomfortable because I thought Amy needed to be in A&E so she could be assessed and sutured if necessary. To some extent, all of this 'paralysed' me and all I could do was watch (it was almost like slow motion) Deb interact with Amy, feeling very helpless myself. At the time, it also made me feel guilty because, as a second-year student, I felt I should have been able to help.

However, being 'rooted to the spot' turned out to have a significant advantage for my learning and my future practice. I watched Deb clean up Amy's wounds, while inspecting them for severity, applying a couple of steri-strips to one of the wounds (there were four wounds in total, all superficial). Most significantly, I listened to Deb as she did this. She was calm and reassuring as she spoke to Amy, asking how she was feeling, what had set this off, what alternative coping approaches (if any) she had tried before cutting, and whether she needed to talk to someone. She also asked Amy if she had been having 'dark' thoughts such as wanting to die, or if any other thoughts had troubled her. This really shocked me at first because I thought Deb would put ideas into Amy's head by asking these sorts of questions. It didn't; in fact, the conversation between Amy and Deb was natural, kind and nurturing – there was clearly trust and rapport between the two. Amy told Deb that some messages on Snapchat had got to her and she had just 'lost it'. She didn't want to die but didn't know what to do when emotional pain came down hard on her. Amy was calmer after about 15 minutes and Deb asked her if she wanted to go home or remain in school. Amy said she preferred to remain in school, so Deb arranged for her to do some classwork in a private side room near the nurse's office. Deb asked me if I would sit outside this side room, just so that Amy had someone near her and that she (Deb) would be just on the other side of the corridor if I needed her. I agreed to do this, but it did panic me a bit in case Amy started cutting again. However, she didn't, and she got on with doing some 'creative writing' classwork. I also did some biosciences revision while sitting outside Amy's room, occasionally checking with Amy that she was OK. Amy said she was, but that she wanted me to stay near her as it was nice knowing someone was there.

At the end of the school day, Deb called me in for a 'debrief'. She explained that she once would have reacted like I had, but added that she had received training in dealing with common mental health problems in schools and this had given her confidence to deal with situations like Amy's. This made me feel a lot better, knowing Deb was once like me. Deb also said that skilled practitioners can manage most self-harm outside of an emergency or mental health setting (though she also made the point that sometimes there are real emergencies like overdosing on medicines), but it requires empathy, kindness and good communication skills. Deb said I already had those qualities but, like her, needed to build up my confidence. This made me feel even better and I started to think again about the kids who come into the paediatric wards who have mental health problems that we all tend to ignore because, to be honest, we are scared of doing or saying the wrong thing.

After this event, I started to read around the topic of children and young people's mental health and, at Deb's suggestion, made some contact with the local mental health service, who invited me to come and talk to the mental health nurses there. I'm thinking about having a formal placement in the children's mental health service as my elective next year and perhaps even doing my dissertation on the topic.

In summary, I have realised that an event where you feel powerless, paralysed and perhaps even inept can – with the right support – turn out be a great learning experience.

Discussion of task

The reflection corresponds to many elements of the reflective models (Borton, 1970; Gibbs, 1988, Johns, 2009) discussed earlier in the chapter. There is:

- **Description** of a particular situation (placement in a secondary school) and the feelings that arose in the student ('wasn't really looking forward to it', 'unnerved me'). There is then a description of a critical incident (self-harming) and the student's immediate reaction to and feelings about the incident (instinct to intervene, feeling uncomfortable and inadequate).

- Insightful **analysis** and **evaluation** of the outcomes of the incident itself, the actions of a more experienced colleague, and, importantly, the opportunity the situation affords for observation and reflection. What initially seemed like a negative – feeling paralysed and helpless – comes to be recognised as a positive – an opportunity to really see what's going on and to think about it objectively: 'being rooted to the spot turned out to have a significant advantage for my learning and future practice'. The writing moves between description of the treatment process and analysis of the student's feelings and developing understanding. She is able to identify her own assumptions, in particular about what kind of conversation is acceptable with such a patient, and explain how these assumptions are challenged by what she experiences.

- Effective **analysis** of the **follow-up** to the incident and the **learning experience** – talking to the experienced colleague about what happened and how certain feelings and reactions might have originated and can be effectively managed.

- **Implications for future practice**: reading around relevant issues, contact with mental health services, a possible placement and dissertation related to this area of nursing.

The language of reflection

Writing reflectively requires command of a particular style of writing, which is in some ways different from the style of writing you will be asked to use in other critical essays.

Reflection

What do you notice about the type of language used in the reflections you have studied in the previous section?

Discussion of reflective language analysis

Reflective writing is characterised by a number of features:

CROSS
REFERENCE

Appendix 2,
Verb forms
in English

- A range of tenses, eg the past tense (simple, continuous, perfect) to describe the incident or experience ('I spent most of my time'; 'this unnerved me'; 'she had been self-harming'); the present tense (simple, continuous, perfect) to describe current feelings and beliefs ('I prefer to work with younger children'; 'I'm thinking about having'; 'I've realised'); the future tense to describe planned action ('I think I'll be'; 'I'm going to contact');

- A slightly conversational tone ('I wasn't really looking forward to'; 'she had just 'lost it'');

- The first person pronoun ('my last placement'; 'I started to read around the topic');

- Words and phrases connected to different aspects of reflection as outlined in the various models (see the next task).

Task

Identifying useful words and phrases

Match the headings (1–7) to the sets (A–G) of phrases below, taken from the previous reflective essay.

1) Reflection on current knowledge and attitudes;

2) Describing feelings;

3) Describing reactions to a situation or incident;

4) Explaining feelings and reactions;

5) Highlighting important points;

6) Signalling how the situation or event has challenged previous thinking;

7) Impact on practice.

A (note the underlined expressions)

This unnerved me at first <u>as</u> I don't really know enough about mental health problems in children and young people.

I tend to ignore or avoid kids who come into the paediatric wards with these problems <u>because</u> I don't know what to do with them.

My immediate reaction was to call for an ambulance <u>as</u> I thought this was clearly a medical emergency.

This made me uncomfortable <u>because</u> I thought Amy needed to be in A&E <u>so</u> she could be assessed and sutured if necessary.

It also made me feel guilty <u>because</u>, as a second-year student, I felt I should have been able to help.

This really shocked me at first <u>because</u> I thought Deb could put ideas into Amy's head by asking these sorts of questions.

B

I wasn't really looking forward to…

I prefer…

I thought…

[I was] feeling very helpless myself.

C

One of the things that struck me immediately was…

This unnerved me.

My immediate reaction was to…

This made me uncomfortable.

All of this 'paralysed' me.

All I could do was watch.

It was almost like slow motion.

It made me feel guilty.

This really shocked me at first.

It did panic me.

This made me feel a lot/even better.

D

At Deb's suggestion, [I] made some contact with…

I'm thinking about…

E

I don't really know enough about…

I don't know what to do with…

I tend to ignore…

I don't know what to do with…

F

Most significantly,…

In fact,…

There was clearly…

G

[This] turned out to have a significant advantage for my learning and my future practice.

I started to think again about…

After this event I started to…

I have realised…

Top tips

Language bank

Make a note of language which will help you to signal and organise the different aspects of your reflection, perhaps adding phrases to a diagram of the reflective model you are using (see Figure 2.3 as an example). Start with the phrases in Figure 2.3 and Table 2.1 below, which add to and expand on the language discussed in the previous task.

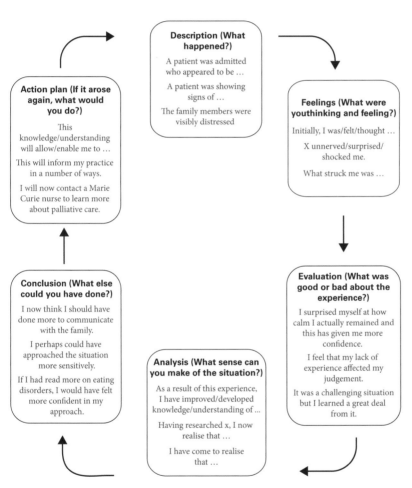

Description (What happened?)

A patient was admitted who appeared to be …

A patient was showing signs of …

The family members were visibly distressed

Feelings (What were you thinking and feeling?)

Initially, I was/felt/thought …

X unnerved/surprised/shocked me.

What struck me was …

Evaluation (What was good or bad about the experience?)

I surprised myself at how calm I actually remained and this has given me more confidence.

I feel that my lack of experience affected my judgement.

It was a challenging situation but I learned a great deal from it.

Analysis (What sense can you make of the situation?)

As a result of this experience, I have improved/developed knowledge/understanding of …

Having researched x, I now realise that …

I have come to realise that …

Conclusion (What else could you have done?)

I now think I should have done more to communicate with the family.

I perhaps could have approached the situation more sensitively.

If I had read more on eating disorders, I would have felt more confident in my approach.

Action plan (If it arose again, what would you do?)

This knowledge/understanding will allow/enable me to …

This will inform my practice in a number of ways.

I will now contact a Marie Curie nurse to learn more about palliative care.

Figure 2.3: An example of a reflective model with language cues added

Table 2.1: The language of reflection

Reflection on current/previous knowledge and attitudes			
I	don't know/understand much/enough about … tend to …		
Prior to this, Previously,	I	had thought that … hadn't been aware of …	

Describing feelings		
(Initially,)	I	was … felt/was feeling … thought …

Describing reactions to a situation or incident	
X	unnerved me surprised me shocked me made me panic made me nervous/uncomfortable/guilty struck me as …
My immediate reaction was to …	
One of the things that What Something that	struck me immediately was … surprised me was … shocked me was …

Highlighting important points			
For me, the most	important significant useful	occurrence event issue	was …
Significantly, … Importantly, … Crucially, … In fact, … Clearly, …			

Signalling how the situation or event has challenged previous thinking				
As a result of this experience, Subsequently,	I have	improved developed improved enhanced	my	knowledge of … understanding of … skills in … ability to …

Having	analysed discussed read researched	x,	I now	feel … know … understand …
I have	realised that … come to realise that … begun to understand …			

Impact on practice			
This	knowledge understanding	will	allow me to … enable me to … inform my practice

Top tips

Beating writer's block!

Sometimes, you may find yourself staring at a blank page, not quite knowing how to start. Don't worry too much about this – you are not alone; it happens to everyone from time to time. The important thing is to have strategies to overcome this writer's block. One thing that can help is to actually start with some key phrases, such as those given in the previous sections, and use these to prompt your own ideas. **The meaningful nature of many of these phrases will also help you to shape your ideas in a more critical way.**

Summary

This chapter has explored the concepts of 'reflection' and 'reflective practice' and their place in critical thinking. It has presented key models of reflective practice and provided opportunities to analyse and evaluate them so that you can determine if and how they will support your own reflective practice. It has highlighted the key distinction between reflection *in* and reflection *on* practice. It has discussed the importance of reflecting on your learning and emphasised the key role of feedback. The chapter has also introduced the important concept of 'clinical supervision'. Finally, it has provided some linguistic tools to help you write reflectively.

References

Borton, T (1970) *Reach, touch and teach: student concerns and process education.* London: Hutchinson.

Gibbs, G (1988) *Learning by doing: a guide to teaching and learning methods.* Oxford: Further Education Unit, Oxford Polytechnic.

Johns, C (2009) *Becoming a reflective practitioner*. 3rd ed. Chichester: Wiley.

Kolb, D, Rubin, I and Osland, J (1991) *Organisational behaviour: an experiential approach*. 5th ed. London: Prentice-Hall International.

NMC (2002) *Supporting nurses and midwives through lifelong learning*. London: NMC.

Pryjmachuk, S (2011) The capable mental health nurse, in Pryjmachuk, S (ed) *Mental health nursing: an evidence-based introduction*. London: Sage, pp. 42–72.

Schön, D (1987) *Educating the reflective practitioner: towards a new design for teaching and learning in the professions*. San Francisco: Jossey-Bass.

Tennant, M. (1997) *Psychology and adult learning*. 2nd ed. London: Routledge.

Chapter 3
Critical reading

Learning outcomes

After reading this chapter you will:

- be able to select academic sources for assignments which are both credible and relevant;

- understand how to engage critically with sources;

- know how to analyse and evaluate arguments and evidence in sources effectively.

In order to complete assignments at university, you will be required to access the literature relevant to your discipline, mostly in the form of textbooks and academic journals. This chapter guides you towards understanding which sources are suitable for the task in hand. It discusses how to engage critically with the literature, how to go about analysing and evaluating the arguments and evidence presented so that you can develop and support your own position in oral and written assignments.

Selecting sources for an assignment

A university assignment, whether it is an academic essay or presentation, is, in many ways, an account of your own critical journey through the literature as you form your position with regard to a particular topic or issue. In academia, this position is often known as your 'stance'.

Your stance is expressed through your argument, and a good argument must draw on and engage with sources that both have credibility in an academic context and are directly relevant to the assignment task or question in hand.

Top tips

Identifying possible sources

Textbooks can be a useful starting point. They can provide an overview of a discipline (eg mental health nursing) or a topic (eg treatments for depression), outlining and illustrating current ideas, beliefs and evidence. They may also summarise the way in which knowledge and understanding in that area has evolved over time, pinpointing any changes in direction regarding the main issues or debates.

CROSS REFERENCE

Studying for your Nursing Degree, Chapter 5, Academic resources: technology and the library, The university library

Journal articles often advance a particular position and argument. This is usually based on a piece of primary research carried out by the authors, but it could also be built around a systematic review of major studies conducted by others. Note that journal articles, which have been subject to a review by an expert panel of referees, are considered to be more academic than articles in periodicals, which tend to be chosen by the editor. Note also that there is a hierarchy of journals and periodicals, with some carrying more weight than others. Influential journals have what is known as a high **impact factor** (Garfield, 2006), and, the more you progress in your studies, the more you will be expected to draw on these weightier journals. Your university library will help you to identify and access appropriate journals by providing access to databases which are important in nursing, such as CINAHL (Cumulative Index of Nursing and Allied Health Literature), MEDLINE, EMBASE and PsycINFO. You can usually access these databases through electronic interfaces such as OVID, EBSCO, ProQuest and PubMed.

Top tips

Reading efficiently

There are limits on the time you can devote to reading, so it is very important to read efficiently. In order to decide if an article will be relevant, you might want to work your way down the list below, putting the article aside as soon as it seems that it may not be relevant to the task, thereby saving precious reading time:

1) the title;
2) the abstract or summary;
3) the keywords (if included);
4) the introduction;
5) the conclusion;
6) the whole article.

Note that a well-written title and abstract may give you all the information you need in the first instance.

Selecting credible sources

In order to assess the *credibility* and *authority* of a source, you should pose a set of critical questions:

- Who wrote/created it? Is the author an academic authority in the field? If an organisation, what type of organisation is it? (A respected professional body, the government, a charity, a corporation?)
- Is it published by a reputable academic publisher/journal?
- What is the author's purpose in writing? (To inform, argue a particular position, sell products?)

- Who is the intended reader or listener? (Students, other scholars, potential customers?)
- Is this source cited by other credible scholars?
- Is it a recent publication? Is this fact relevant/important – do later publications draw on new evidence, or advance the argument in any way, for example?
- What is the scope of the work? Is it comprehensive, or is it limited in some way?

Selecting relevant sources

It is important to be able to establish that a source has credibility in an academic sense; however, to be of any use to you in an assignment, a source must also be *relevant*. It is not enough that a source is merely connected to the topic in hand; relevance can only be established with precise reference to your precise **purpose** in writing or presenting, and this entails careful analysis of the assignment task or question. This initial 'unpacking' of the task requires careful, *critical* reading.

Task

Unpacking the task

Look at the following Level 5 essay-writing tasks and identify the following (discussed later in the chapter):

- the general **topic**;
- the particular **focus** of the assignment;
- any **instruction words** which tell you how to **approach** the assignment.

A

Outline current practices on handwashing in healthcare settings and critically evaluate the extent to which handwashing practices can reduce hospital-acquired infection.

B

Critically explore the unique contribution that registered nurses might make to the effective care and support of older people with long-term health conditions.

Task

Assessing the relevance of journal articles

Look at the following extracts (title; summary; keywords) from journal articles and decide if and in what way they might relate to the essays in the previous task.

CROSS REFERENCE

Academic Writing and Referencing for your Nursing Degree, Chapter 1, Academic writing: text, process and criticality, The writing process, Approaching a writing assignment

CROSS REFERENCE

Academic Writing and Referencing for your Nursing Degree, Chapter 1, Academic writing: text, process and criticality, The writing process, Analysing a writing assignment

CROSS REFERENCE

Appendix 1, Academic levels at university

CROSS REFERENCE

Discussion of task: assessing the relevance of journal articles

1)

Title

'My five moments for hand hygiene': a user-centred design approach to understand, train, monitor and report hand hygiene

Summary

Hand hygiene is a core element of patient safety for the prevention of healthcare-associated infections and the spread of antimicrobial resistance. Its promotion represents a challenge that requires a multi-modal strategy using a clear, robust and simple conceptual framework. The World Health Organization First Global Patient Safety Challenge 'Clean Care is Safer Care' has expanded educational and promotional tools developed initially for the Swiss national hand hygiene campaign for worldwide use. Development methodology involved a user-centred design approach incorporating strategies of human factors engineering, cognitive behaviour science and elements of social marketing, followed by an iterative prototype test phase within the target population. This research resulted in a concept called 'My five moments for hand hygiene'. It describes the fundamental reference points for healthcare workers (HCWs) in a time–space framework and designates the moments when hand hygiene is required to effectively interrupt microbial transmission during the care sequence. The concept applies to a wide range of patient care activities and healthcare settings. It proposes a unified vision for trainers, observers and HCWs that should facilitate education, minimize inter-individual variation and resource use, and increase adherence. 'My five moments for hand hygiene' bridges the gap between scientific evidence and daily health practice and provides a solid basis to understand, teach, monitor and report hand-hygiene practices.

Keywords

Hand hygiene; Healthcare-associated infections; Patient safety; Healthcare workers

(Sax et al, 2007)

2)

Title

Use of a Patient Hand Hygiene Protocol to Reduce Hospital-Acquired Infections and Improve Nurses' Hand Washing

Abstract

Background Critically ill patients are at marked risk of hospital-acquired infections, which increase patients' morbidity and mortality.

Registered nurses are the main healthcare providers of physical care, including hygiene to reduce and prevent hospital-acquired infections, for hospitalized critically ill patients.

Objective To investigate a new patient hand hygiene protocol designed to reduce hospital-acquired infection rates and improve nurses' hand-washing compliance in an intensive care unit.

Methods A preexperimental study design was used to compare 12-month rates of 2 common hospital-acquired infections, central catheter-associated bloodstream infection and catheter-associated urinary tract infection, and nurses' hand-washing compliance measured before and during use of the protocol.

Results Reductions in 12-month infection rates were reported for both types of infections, but neither reduction was statistically significant. Mean 12-month nurse hand-washing compliance also improved, but not significantly.

Conclusions A hand hygiene protocol for patients in the intensive care unit was associated with reductions in hospital-acquired infections and improvements in nurses' hand-washing compliance. Prevention of such infections requires continuous quality improvement efforts to monitor lasting effectiveness as well as investigation of strategies to eliminate these infections.

(Fox et al, 2015)

3)

Title

Long-Term Care and a Good Quality of Life: Bringing Them Closer Together

Abstract
Long-term care policies and programs in the United States suffer from a major flaw: They are balanced toward a model of nursing home care that, regardless of its technical quality, tends to be associated with a poor quality of life for consumers. This article proposes quality-of-life domains – namely, security, comfort, meaningful activity, relationships, enjoyment, dignity, autonomy, privacy, individuality, spiritual well-being, and functional competence. It argues that these kinds of quality-of-life outcomes are minimized in current quality assessment and given credence only after health and safety outcomes are considered. Five trends are reviewed that might lead to a more consumer-centered emphasis on

quality of life: the disability rights movement, the emphasis on consumer direction, the growth of assisted living, increasing attention to physical environments, and efforts to bring about culture change in nursing homes. Building on these trends, the article concludes with strategies to move beyond current stalemates and polarized arguments toward forms of long-term care that are more compatible with a good quality of life.

Keywords
Public policy, Nursing homes, Home care, Assisted living

(Kane, 2001)

4)

Title

A critical literature review exploring the challenges of delivering effective palliative care to older people with dementia

Abstract

Aim This paper considers the challenges of delivering effective palliative care to older people with dementia and the possible strategies to overcome barriers to end-of-life care in these patients.

Background In UK alone, approximately 100 000 people with dementia die each year and as the number of older people increases, dementia is set to become even more prevalent. Dementia is a progressive terminal illness for which there is currently no cure. Patients dying with dementia have significant health care needs and in recent years it has been recognised that palliative care should be made available to everyone regardless of diagnosis, as this improves comfort and quality of life. Despite this, patients dying with dementia are often still not given access to palliative care services.

Method A review of English language literature published after 1996 to the present day relating to older people with dementia during the terminal phase of their illness.

Results Twenty-nine articles met inclusion criteria for the review. Most originated from North America and UK and were mostly quantitative in nature. Four key themes were identified: difficulties associated with diagnosing the terminal phase of the illness (prognostication); issues relating to communication; medical interventions; and the appropriateness of palliative care intervention.

Conclusions This review reinforces the importance of providing appropriate palliative care to individuals suffering from end-stage dementia and identifies some of the barriers to extending such specialist palliative care provision.

Relevance to practice There is an urgent need to improve palliative care provision for older people with end-stage dementia and, in addition, more research is required on the needs of patients entering the terminal phase of dementia to assist the allocation of appropriate resources and training to ensure quality and equality in the provision of end-of-life care.

(Birch and Draper, 2008)

Discussion of tasks

You first need to think carefully about the words you highlighted earlier in the chapter, related to topic, focus, and instruction:

CROSS REFERENCE

Task, Analysing the task

A

| Instruction words | Topic | Instruction words |

<u>Outline</u> current practices on hand washing in healthcare settings and <u>critically evaluate the extent to which</u> handwashing practices can reduce hospital acquired infection.

Focus

The paper described in Abstract 1 is relevant to this assignment as it is relatively up to date (2007; though you might want to see if there have been updates by the authors), is clearly related to handwashing in healthcare settings, and mentions prevention of infections. It is also likely to be evidence based because the abstract claims that the 'my five moments for hand-hygiene' approach 'bridges the gap between scientific evidence and daily health practice and provides a solid basis to understand, teach, monitor and report hand hygiene practices'.

The paper described in Abstract 2 is also relevant to this assignment for similar reasons and it is more current (2015) than the paper described in Abstract 1. It also helps students with the 'critically evaluate' element of the assignment because not only is it a research-based paper, but the results do not necessarily indicate that a specific handwashing protocol *significantly* reduces infection rates.

B

| Instruction words | Focus |

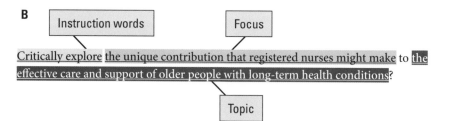

<u>Critically explore</u> the unique contribution that registered nurses might make to the effective care and support of older people with long-term health conditions?

Topic

The paper described in Abstract 3 is a potentially useful source for this assignment, although you would need to ensure that the paper is concerned with registered nurses and not just people who work in nursing homes – remember, the assignment asks about the *unique* contribution of registered nurses. It is also a US paper, so you can demonstrate that you are being critical by noting this and questioning the relevance of papers exploring US healthcare with regard to British healthcare.

The paper described in Abstract 4 is also potentially useful for this assignment, as dementia is clearly a long-term health condition affecting older people. In addition, being a review of the literature, it focuses on the evidence base in this area and so can help you be more critical. However, although the paper talks about *care*, you would need to ensure that it has a focus on or discusses the importance of care that is delivered by registered nurses rather than, say, healthcare assistants, because you would not otherwise be able to explore the *unique* contribution of registered nurses. On the other hand, if it did focus primarily on healthcare assistants' role in the palliative care of older people with dementia and there is evidence that their role is important and effective, you might actually want to argue that registered nurses *do not* make a unique contribution. This would certainly demonstrate that you are being critical and operating at Level 5, which is the level the assignment is set at.

CROSS
REFERENCE

Chapter 4,
Critical writing,
What does it
mean to write
critically?

Engaging critically with sources

The work that you produce on your degree programme should be informed and enhanced by the literature. You should therefore read with an eye to doing more than merely reproducing the ideas and arguments of others in word-for-word notes. Such a 'knowledge-telling' approach (Beirerter and Scardamalia, 1987) could ultimately lead to your own work ending up as a mere 'patchwork' of ideas, and you will probably be criticised for being overly descriptive and uncritical. It is therefore necessary to *engage critically* with the literature, and to adopt a 'knowledge-transforming' approach (Beirerter and Scardamalia, 1987); this means scrutinising and synthesising the ideas, arguments and evidence you encounter as you read, with a view to using them to develop your own position.

Scrutinising

As you note and relate the arguments and evidence you encounter, it is important to scrutinise them, asking questions as you read:

- Is an argument based on sound reasoning?
- Is there sufficient evidence to support the argument?
- Is the evidence credible and convincing?
- Has evidence (or alternative interpretations of evidence) which might counter the argument been given due consideration?

Synthesising

Reading critically means being careful not to look at facts, ideas, arguments, evidence, findings, conclusions etc in isolation. The critical reader is alert to any trends, patterns or relationships which emerge as they read across the literature, and is conscious of anything which may not fit into these. The ideal is to find ways to represent these things in your notes as you encounter them, organising the ideas and evidence you discover, so that you are already preparing to say something about how *you* understand and interpret the current state of knowledge. [In Chapter 4 of *Studying for your Nursing Degree*, there is an example of how note-taking (in this case on treatment pathways for depression) can develop in a focused, critical fashion.]

It is also vital to constantly relate what you find in the literature with your particular context, ie the task or question you are working on.

Telling your research story

As noted earlier, the academic work you produce is in some ways the story of your journey through the literature, an account of how your own thought processes have developed as you encountered, analysed and evaluated the ideas and arguments of scholars in the field. This is the essence of **originality** (and the antithesis of *plagiarism*!), as the journey you have been on is unique to you, and only you can tell this story. This individual and unique **voice** is what makes your essay different from other people's essays. If you approach the reading and writing process with this in mind, your voice should grow to be mature and confident.

CROSS REFERENCE

Studying for your Nursing Degree, Critical thinking, Applying and developing your critical thinking skills, Synthesis of information and ideas

CROSS REFERENCE

Chapter 4, Critical writing, What does it mean to write critically?

Task

> ### Being a critical reader
>
> Read the extracts below (taken from the journal articles introduced earlier in the chapter) and answer the questions. (The questions are aimed at helping you to read critically.)
>
> **A**
>
> #### Practical applications of the model
> A multi-modal approach to hand hygiene promotion has been found to be the most efficient technique to increase patient safety in a sustained way.[8,21,27,56,57] A robust description of the critical moments for hand hygiene is important for the various elements of a multi-modal strategy including training, workplace reminders, ergonomic localisation of hand rub at the point of care, performance assessment by direct observations, and reporting.
>
> (Sax et al, 2007)

Questions

1) What key concepts are introduced in this extract?

2) What do you understand them to mean?

3) In what way are they relevant to essay A (discussed earlier in the chapter)?

B

Most people who reach middle years also can test their generalizations about LTC against the experiences of family members and friends. Reflecting on personal "data" is a good antidote to the hubris of presuming to discuss, let alone measure, a good quality of life for those faced with the realities of LTC and the conditions and circumstances that generated its need. As of this writing, the most vivid part of my database includes the experiences of my father (age 93 and healthy but with encroaching macular degeneration) and my mother (age 86 and functionally limited because of osteoporosis), who are so far managing at home; my mother-in-law, who is experiencing physical and cognitive post-stroke problems in a New York assisted living setting; my maternal aunt, who had intensive and escalating needs for both formal and family care during the 3 months between diagnosis of liver cancer and her death in her own home close to her 80th birthday; a paternal uncle, whose Parkinson's disease limits his functioning drastically, first at home with his wife and now in an assisted living setting in Ontario; a paternal aunt, whose multiple sclerosis necessitated years of in-home care and about 6 years of nursing home care before her death; and other now mostly deceased uncles and aunts and more distant relatives who collectively illustrate a wide variety of chronic illnesses and social circumstances with an admixture of mental health problems and, for a few, Alzheimer's disease. This collection of family stories immediately reveals that one solution cannot fit all. So, too, do findings from a 5-year longitudinal in-depth study of 300 family caregivers (Kane and Penrod 1995; Kane, Reinardy, Penrod, Huck, and Finch 1999), which shows that the dominant tendency in family care (i.e., female, average age in the late 50s) masks the incredible variety that occurs in the real world and the imaginative way ordinary people invent solutions to problems that disability creates in their everyday lives.

(Kane, 2001)

Questions

1) What does the author mean by 'personal data'?

2) What sort of 'evidence' of effective nursing care is the author presenting here?

3) What arguments are made regarding the value of using reflections on personal experiences in understanding and designing nursing care?

4) What might be problematic about using this kind of data?

Discussion of task

A

1) Concept clarification is an essential part of good essay writing. Two key concepts are introduced in this essay: 'multi-modal approach' and 'critical moment'.

2) A multi-modal approach clearly involves a number of elements and these are exemplified in the extract. In the term 'critical moment', critical means 'important'.

3) The extract makes it clear that a multi-modal approach is evidence based. The citations provide evidence of its efficiency. This will inform your own position with regard to the essay task.

B

1) and 2) The author is making a **qualitative** v **quantitative** argument. Qualitative data can involve personal data (experiences; stories), which can offer a different perspective on quality of life compared to quantitative data (numbers; measurements). Note that nursing research often uses a **mixed methods** approach, combining quantitative and qualitative data.

3) By reflecting on personal experiences, the author stresses the point that the experience of each individual requiring care is unique. Thus, when planning care, 'one solution cannot fit all'.

4) Some qualitative data could be seen as anecdotal and its relevance might not be easily generalisable.

CROSS REFERENCE

Studying for your Nursing Degree, Chapter 3, Becoming a member of your academic and professional community, Academic principles, pursuits and practices, Teaching, research and knowledge

Summary

This chapter has guided you in the selection of credible, relevant sources, and suggested ways in which you can engage critically with the literature. It has demonstrated how critical engagement with the literature at the reading stage is necessary in order to develop and support your own arguments when you come to writing essays or presenting work.

Sources of example texts

Birch, D and Draper, J (2008) A critical literature review exploring the challenges of delivering effective palliative care to older people with dementia. *Journal of clinical nursing*, 17(9): 1144–63 [online]. Available at: http://onlinelibrary.wiley.com/doi/10.1111/j.1365-2702.2007.02220.x/full (accessed 5 March 2018).

Fox, C. et al (2015) Use of a patient hand hygiene protocol to reduce hospital-acquired infections and improve nurses' hand washing. *American journal of critical care*, 24: 216–24 [online]. Available at: http://ajcc.aacnjournals.org/content/24/3/216.short (accessed 5 March 2018).

Kane, R (2001) Long-term care and a quality of life: bringing them closer together. *The gerontologist*, 41(3): 293–304 [online]. Available at: https://academic.oup.com/gerontologist/article/41/3/293/632406 (accessed 5 March 2018).

Sax, H. et al (2007) 'My five moments for hand hygiene': a user-centred design approach to understand, train, monitor and report hand hygiene. *Journal of hospital infection*, 67(1): 9–21 [online]. Available at: www.sciencedirect.com/science/article/pii/S0195670107001909 (accessed 5 March 2018).

References

Beirerter, C and Sardamalia, M (1987) *The psychology of written composition*. Hillsdale, NJ: Lawrence Erlbaum.

Garfield, E (2006) The history and meaning of the journal impact factor. *JAMA*, 295(1): 90–3 [online]. Available at: http://garfield.library.upenn.edu/papers/jamajif2006.pdf (accessed 5 March 2018).

Chapter 4
Critical writing

Learning outcomes

After reading this chapter you will:

- understand what it means to write critically;

- have a better understanding of the concepts of voice, stance and argument;

- be better able to express criticality in your writing.

At the beginning of your studies, you will mainly be required to focus on describing and demonstrating your knowledge and understanding of concepts, theories and research in nursing. As you progress through your nursing degree, this knowledge and understanding will need to be increasingly underpinned by **criticality**. This chapter will further explain what criticality means, and then help you to incorporate and express criticality in your writing.

What does it mean to write critically?

As discussed in Chapter 3, Critical reading, it is important to engage critically with the literature as you research the topic of your essay. Writing critically entails making this critical engagement explicit for the reader, and using it as a platform on which to build your own argument, as you accept, reject or suspend judgement on the claims put forward in the literature.

Lecturers often cite a lack of criticality as a reason for low marks. Essays lacking in criticality are usually overly descriptive. This can mean that the writer simply reports what is in the literature, leading to a kind of 'patchwork' of other people's views. When a lecturer reads this kind of writing, they will be asking, 'But where are *you* in all this? What do *you* think now you have learned so much about the views and claims of others?' What they are looking for is your **voice**. It can be difficult to have the confidence to insert your voice in amongst the voices of respected academics and scholars, and it can take time to find and develop your own individual voice. However, it is essential if you are to be a critical writer. Criticality is essentially related to having a clear voice, having something to say, being in possession of an independent viewpoint based on an understanding of the literature and the available evidence. This viewpoint is often called your **stance**, ie your position in relation to the topic. It is not enough to state your position; you need to guide the reader through the thought processes via which you arrived at it and provide an evidence-based rationale to support it. The expression of your stance is your **argument**, the line of reasoning which is the backbone of a critical essay. You should be confident in your argument, but this does not mean being close-minded or rigid. In fact, a strong argument usually possesses significant

CROSS
REFERENCE

*Academic
Writing and
Referencing
for your
Nursing
Degree,*
Chapter 1,
Academic
writing: text,
process and
criticality,
Writing
critically

nuance. A nuanced argument acknowledges strengths, weaknesses and grey areas. It means sometimes qualifying your claims or recognising limitations. Last but not least, in order to make your argument clear, nuanced and persuasive, it is often necessary to use very specific **language** associated with criticality in academic writing (see for example: Biber, 2006; Argent, 2017). This can involve:

- Language which specifically conveys opinion, eg 'this clearly shows', 'unfortunately', 'surprisingly';

- Language which signals understanding of complexity in a situation, eg 'however/although/despite/on the other hand';

- The use of 'summary nouns' (Drummond, 2016) or 'signalling nouns' (Flowerdew, 2003), ie nouns which refer back to something previously mentioned, often signalling an element of opinion or interpretation, eg 'this decisive action', 'these so-called wonder drugs', 'this controversial treatment';

CROSS
REFERENCE

*Academic
Writing and
Referencing
for your
Nursing
Degree,*
Chapter 2,
Coherent
texts and
arguments,
The language
of criticality

- Verbs and other expressions used to report, and often to interpret, what has been said or written, eg 'the consensus is', 'Turner et al advocate a course of antibiotics', 'there is limited evidence in this area';

- The use of language which conveys varying degrees of certainty, especially the use of cautious language to avoid overgeneralisation or unsubstantiated claims, eg 'this appears to be a common symptom', 'there are approximately 10,000 people currently infected', 'this suggests that nurses are…'.

Task

Identifying critical use of language

Identify the language used to convey criticality in the following text extracts.

1) It seems that nurses are under significant pressure to demonstrate that their work improves outcomes, while at the same time being cost effective. In order to meet these challenges, nurses must ensure that their practice is research informed.

2) Midwives may need to develop additional skills when working in rural and remote areas. This could involve skills around the support of teenage mothers and families.

3) In conclusion, there have been a number of recent high-profile cases of abuse involving the elderly or those with learning disabilities. While these almost undoubtedly involve a minority of practitioners, they clearly demonstrate the need for a renewed commitment to patient care and safety throughout the health and social care professions.

4) The limited benefits associated with the use of acupuncture during childbirth should be weighed against the cost of providing this treatment.

5) The authors question the effectiveness of many of the healthcare programmes that have recently been introduced to target the homeless.

Task

Identifying critical essay writing

Look again at the essay title from Chapter 3.

A

Outline current practices on handwashing in healthcare settings and critically evaluate the extent to which handwashing practices can reduce healthcare-acquired infection.

1) In what ways does this essay title require students to engage critically with the topic and with the literature?

2) Which parts of the essay will be the least/most descriptive?

3) Read the student essay below and find examples of critical writing.

4) Can you find examples of language use which signal the student's criticality?

5) Are there any ways in which the student could have been more critical?

Introduction

Technological advances have greatly improved the treatment of many diseases and disorders. However, these advances are often undermined by the transmission of infections within healthcare settings, in particular, those resulting from antimicrobial-resistant strains of disease-causing microorganisms, which are now endemic in many healthcare environments (Allegranzi et al, 2011; Loveday et al, 2014). In 2009, healthcare-associated infection (HCAI) affected 5–15 per cent of hospitalised patients in the developed world (WHO, 2009). This figure rises to 9–37 per cent for critically ill patients in intensive care units (ICUs), who are particularly susceptible to HCAI. The most frequently occurring HCAIs affecting these patients are urinary tract infection, surgical site infection, bloodstream infection and pneumonia (WHO, 2009). Studies report higher rates in developing countries, although, according to the World Health Organization, this data, mostly collected in single hospital studies, is a less reliable indicator of wider trends. The huge personal, social and financial costs associated with HCAI have led to a growing public awareness of the threat, and of the need for urgent solutions.

Epidemiological evidence indicates that hand-transmission is a major contributing factor in the acquisition and spread of HCAI (Loveday et al, 2014). For this reason, healthcare workers' hand hygiene is traditionally considered as the single most important factor in the reduction of HCAI (Gould et al, 2017). Studies on the effects of handwashing protocols in healthcare settings date back to the mid-1800s (WHO, 2009), but it was not until 2001 that the first national evidence-based guidelines for preventing HCAI in NHS hospitals, including hand hygiene as one of its principal interventions, were introduced by the Department of Health in the UK (Loveday et al, 2014).

This essay will begin by outlining current handwashing practices in healthcare settings, with particular reference to national NHS guidelines. It will then examine current evidence, including systematic reviews, in order to critically evaluate the extent to which particular practices can reduce HCAI. The main focus will be on the effectiveness of cleaning agents and the issue of compliance. It will conclude with suggestions on recommendations for nursing practice and suggestions regarding which areas can be usefully investigated further.

Current guidelines on hand hygiene
Globally, one of the most influential frameworks for training, auditing and feedback regarding hand-hygiene practice is the World Health Organization's (WHO) 'Five moments for hand hygiene' (Sax et al, 2007). It has been adopted in many countries, often with local modifications. In the UK, NHS guidelines for preventing HCAIs, developed by a nurse-led team of researchers and specialists, were first introduced in 2001, and updated in 2007 (Loveday et al, 2014). These national guidelines are evidence-based 'broad principles of best practice' which need to be integrated into local contexts (Loveday et al, 2014, p 51). Evidence-based guidelines must be carefully monitored and frequently updated as new evidence and technologies emerge, and Loveday et al, commissioned by the Department of Health, reviewed the existing evidence and found that the 2007 guidelines remained 'robust, relevant and appropriate' on the whole (2014, p 51). However, they did put forward a number of new recommendations, as well as proposals for adjustments to existing recommendations.

The standard principles governing the guidelines are based around five distinct interventions (Loveday et al, 2014):

- hospital environment hygiene;
- hand hygiene;
- use of personal protective equipment;
- safe use and disposal of sharps;
- principles of asepsis.

This essay focuses on the second of these: hand hygiene. The current national guidelines on handwashing, as outlined by Loveday et al (2014), are summarised below.

The guidelines require that healthcare workers:

- decontaminate their hands with soap and water or, in some circumstances, an alcohol-based hand rub (ABHR), at key points such as before and after each episode of patient contact or care;
- wear short sleeves, remove all hand jewellery, keep fingernails short, clean and free from polish or false nails, and cover cuts and abrasions with waterproof dressings;
- employ effective handwashing techniques involving three stages: preparation, washing and rinsing, and drying;
- regularly use an emollient hand cream to offset potential skin irritation from decontamination products;
- have access to alcohol-based hand rub at the point of care;
- have access to regular training on hand hygiene.

New recommendations by Loveday et al focus on *education and promotion* of the guidelines:

- 'Local programmes of education, social marketing, and auditing and feedback should be refreshed regularly and promoted by senior managers and clinicians to maintain focus, engage staff and produce sustainable levels of compliance.'

(Loveday et al, 2014, p 54)

It is notable that other additions to the guidelines focus on wider *inclusivity*, with requirements that patients and relatives be included in the process:

- Patients and relatives should be provided with information regarding the need for hand hygiene and how to keep their own hands clean.
- Patients should be offered the opportunity to clean their hands at key points such as before meals or after using the toilet, with appropriate products being made available.

The guidelines are evidence based and set out broad principles, but within these, there are still some areas of doubt, in particular, regarding the comparative effectiveness of cleaning agents and the best way to achieve compliance among healthcare workers.

Cleaning agents

The evidence regarding the effectiveness of particular handwashing agents shows no clear pattern. Turner et al (2010) reported that 65 per cent of ethanol hand sanitisers were more effective in removing Rhinovirus than soap and water. However, Grayson et al (2009) and Oughton et al (2009) reported that soap and water was more effective than ABHR for H1N1 influenza virus and *C. difficile*, respectively. Other studies report no significant difference. The review of national guidelines conducted by Loveday et al (2014) found that, overall, there is no compelling evidence to support a particular type of antiseptic handwashing agent, or to suggest that the use of these is preferable to liquid soap. They conclude that it is not possible to establish a causal relationship between ABHR and reductions in HCAIs. In fact, ABHR is reported to be ineffective in some situations, and even in studies which appear to suggest the superior effectiveness of ABHR, closer investigation often reveals that its use is in fact only one of a number of interventions.

Compliance

Loveday et al (2014) stress the importance of compliance in their updated guidelines, but compliance is notoriously difficult to assess: self-reporting can lead to overestimation (Biran et al, 2008), and the presence of an observer can lead to biased results (Pedersen et al, 1986; Ram et al, 2010). It is therefore necessary to treat reported figures on compliance with caution. However, available figures suggest that healthcare workers often comply poorly with handwashing guidelines (Allegranzi and Pitter, 2009). One recent systematic review estimated compliance to be between 48 and 72 per cent in high-income countries and between 5 and 25 per cent in low-income countries (Freeman et al, 2014), with an overall mean of only 19 per cent.

There is some evidence that clear handwashing guidelines and protocols can improve nurses' compliance with hand-hygiene recommendations (Sax et al, 2007; Fox et al, 2015). The systematic implementation of particular guidelines or protocols is known as a *multi-modal approach*. Possibly the most well known of these is the WHO's 'My five moments for hand hygiene', which, according to Sax et al, 'bridges the gap between scientific evidence and daily health practice and provides a solid basis to understand, teach, monitor and report hand hygiene practices' (Sax et al, 2007, pp 9–10).

However, according to the most recent Cochrane systematic review on hand hygiene (Gould et al, 2017), the best way to achieve compliance with current recommendations on hand hygiene is yet to be established. Both single-intervention strategies and combinations of strategies, many based on WHO recommendations, have been shown to improve hand-hygiene compliance in many healthcare settings. However, it remains unclear which strategy or combination of strategies is most effective in a particular context (Gould et al, 2017).

Conclusion

In conclusion, clear handwashing guidelines and protocols are provided in many healthcare settings, including the NHS, and these may make a significant contribution towards the prevention of HCAI as part of an overall hygiene strategy if they are strictly implemented, and regularly monitored and updated. The evidence indicates that cleanliness itself is more important than the method of cleaning; much research has been conducted on cleaning agents yet no clear winner has emerged. However, compliance emerges as a key factor, and it seems that clear guidelines and protocols can go some way to improving this, although it remains unclear which particular approaches bring most success. While organisational action is vital, it is also important that nurses and other healthcare workers take personal responsibility and closely follow patient safety aspects of the Code (2015), especially 19: 'Be aware of, and reduce as far as possible, any potential for harm associated with your practice'.

References

Allegranzi, B and Pitter, D (2009) Role of hand hygiene in healthcare-associated infection prevention. *The journal of hospital infection*, 73: 305–15.

Allegranzi, B et al (2011) *Report on the burden of endemic healthcare-associated infection worldwide*. Geneva: WHO Press.

Biran, A, Rabie, T, Schmidt, W, Juvekar, S, Hirve, S and Curtis, V (2008) Comparing the performance of indicators of hand-washing practices in rural Indian households. *Tropical medicine and international health*, 13: 278–85.

Fox, C, Wavra, T, Drake, D, Mulligan, D, Bennett, Y, Nelson, C, Kirkwood, P, Jones, L and Bader, M (2015) Use of a patient hand hygiene protocol to reduce hospital-acquired infections and improve nurses' hand washing. *American journal of critical care*, 24(3): 216–24.

Freeman, M, Stocks, M, Cumming, M, Jeandron, A, Higgins, J, Wolf, J, Pruss-Uston, A, Bonjour, S, Hunter, P, Fewtrell, L and Curtis V (2014) Hygiene and health: systematic review of handwashing practices worldwide and update of health effects. *Tropical medicine and international health*, 19(8): 906–16.

Gould, D, Moralejo, D, Drey, N, Chudleigh, J and Taljaard, M (2017) Interventions to improve hand hygiene compliance in patient care. *Cochrane database of systematic reviews*, Issue 9, Art. no.: CD005186.

Grayson, M, Melvani, S, Druce, J, Barr, I, Ballard, S, Johnson, P, Mastorakos, T and Birch, C (2009) Efficacy of soap and water and alcohol-based hand-rub preparations against live H1N1 influenza virus on the hands of human volunteers. *Clinical infectious diseases*, 48(3): 285–91.

Loveday, H, Wilson, J, Pratt, R, Golsorkhi, M, Tingle, A, Bak, A, Browne, J, Prieto, J and Wilcox, M (2014) National evidence-based guidelines for preventing healthcare-assocaited infections in NHS hospitals in England. *The official journal of the healthcare infection society*, 86(1): S1–S70.

Nursing and Midwifery Council (2015) The Code: professional standards of practice and behaviour for nurses and Midwives [online]. Available at: www.nmc.org.uk/globalassets/sitedocuments/nmc-publications/nmc-code.pdf (accessed 5 March 2018).

Oughton, M T, Loo, V G, Dendukuri, N, Fenn, S and Libman, M D (2009) Hand hygiene with soap and water is superior to alcohol rub and antiseptic wipes for removal of clostridium difficile. *Infect control hosp epidemiol*, 30(10): 939–44.

Pedersen, D, Keithly, S and Brady, K (1986) Effects of an observer on conformity to handwashing norm. *Perceptual and motor skills*, 62: 169–70.

Ram P, et al (2010) Is structured observation a valid technique to measure handwashing behavior? Use of acceleration sensors embedded in soap to assess reactivity to structured observation. *The American journal of tropical medicine and hygiene*, 83: 1070–6.

Sax, H, Allegranzi, B, Uçkay, I, Larson, E, Boyce, J and Pittet, D (2007) 'My five moments for hand hygiene': A user-centred design approach to understand, train, monitor and report hand hygiene. *Journal of hospital infection*, 67(1): 9–21 [online]. Available at: www.sciencedirect.com/science/article/pii/S0195670107001909 (accessed 5 March 2018).

Turner, R, Fuls, J and Rodgers, N (2010) Effectiveness of hand sanitizers with and without organic acids for the removal of rhinovirus from hands. *Antimicrobe agents chemother*, 54, 1363–4.

World Health Organization (2009) WHO guidelines on hand hygiene in health care [online]. Available at: www.who.int/gpsc/5may/tools/9789241597906/en/ (accessed 5 March 2018).

Task

Identifying opportunities for criticality

Look again at the essay title from Chapter 3.

B

Critically explore the unique contribution that registered nurses might make to the effective care and support of older people with long-term health conditions.

 1) Look at the student's essay outline and notes below and decide which parts will be the most/least descriptive/analytical and evaluative.

2) Identify opportunities for critical engagement with the topic and the literature.

Introduction

- Define long-term conditions.

- Give contextual background particularly relating to long-term conditions in older people (most common = diabetes, chronic obstructive pulmonary disease, hypertension, heart disease, etc). Dementia could be included?

- The focus is on those who care for/support older people with LTCs. Stress that the assignment needs to focus on registered nurses – to do this probably need to discuss other workers who do 'nursing' but are not nurses (healthcare assistants, care workers, support workers, etc).

- Identify any relevant policy/government documents.

- Explain how I intend to answer the question posed (signpost).

Main section

- Determine what would be deemed to be 'effective' care – suspect things like quality of life and fewer hospital or GP appointments would be good outcomes.

- Likely self-management would play a big role here. (In dementia, may be relatives/carers who do most of self-management.)

- Look for literature on the extent to which registered nurses support self-management. Probably best to look at who supports self-management in general in older people and see if registered nurses feature highly; if not, could argue registered nurses don't make unique contribution.

- Outline key things registered nurses can do that other care workers can't (assessments, meds management, possibly even prescribing) when trying to argue for *unique* contribution.

Summary/Conclusion

- Bring it all together for the reader, perhaps summarising the previous section in a paragraph.

- Draw a strong conclusion relating to registered nurses' *unique* contribution (or not, as the case may be).

- Think about implications for future practice/changing future practice.

Summary

This chapter has explored what it means to write critically. It has discussed the place of voice, stance and argument in critical writing, and highlighted the importance of careful language use. It has demonstrated the characteristics of critical writing with reference to examples of typical student writing. It has thus provided tools which will help you to write critically in your essays.

References

Argent, S (2017) The language of critical thinking [online]. Available at: www.baleap. org/event/eap-northcritical-thinking (accessed 5 March 2018).

Biber, D (2006) Stance in spoken and written university registers. *Journal of English for academic purposes*, 5(2): 97–116.

Drummond, A (2016) An investigation of noun frequencies in cohesive nominal groups. *Journal of second language teaching and research*, 5(1): 62–88.

Flowerdew, J (2003) Signalling nouns in discourse. *English for specific purposes*, 22(4): 329–46.

Appendix 1
Academic levels at university

UNDERGRADUATE STUDY			
England, Wales, Northern Ireland	**Scotland**	**Award**	**Notes**
Level 4	Level 7	Certificate of Higher Education (CertHE)	
Level 5	Level 8	Diploma of Higher Education (DipHE) Foundation Degree (FdD)	Up until 2010, minimum academic qualification for nurses
Level 6	Level 9	Ordinary Bachelor Degree eg BSc Nursing	Minimum academic qualification for nurses and midwives; common exit point in Scotland
	Level 10	Bachelor Degree with Honours eg BSc (Hons) in Nursing Studies, BNurs (Hons), BMidwif (Hons)	Usual academic qualification for nurses and midwives in England, Wales and Northern Ireland
Postgraduate study			
Level 7	Level 11	Masters Degree, eg MSc, MA, MPhil Postgraduate Certificate or Diploma (PGCert; PGDip)	Minimum academic qualification for Advanced Practitioners
Level 8	Level 12	Research Doctorate (PhD) Professional Doctorate eg DNurs, MD, ClinPsychD	Recommended qualification for Advanced Practitioners who are Nurse Consultants

Appendix 2
Verb forms in English

As you write, your choice of verb form will provide important information for your reader as regards when something occurred, how this occurrence is or should be viewed, and how it relates to the current time and context.

Verbs in English possess three important elements:

- **tense** (past, present, future), indicating the time or period in which something occurred;
- **aspect** (simple, continuous, perfect), indicating how the occurrence is perceived;
- **voice** (active, passive), indicating whether the focus is on the action itself or on the agency of the action (ie the person or thing doing it).

Some examples of common uses in academic writing are presented below with explanations as regards usage.

1) Present simple and continuous

The present simple is used for facts:

> Most people **feel** anxiety at some point in their lives.
> The adrenal glands **are found** just above the kidneys.

In the first sentence, it is important that we know who feels something (people), so the active voice is used. In the second sentence, it is the location which is important, not a hypothetical 'finder', hence the passive voice. The passive is common in academic writing as it allows for an impersonal style, eg 'it is believed that' rather than 'people believe'.

The present continuous describes current actions or developments:

> I **am** currently **working** in a paediatric ward.
> Attitudes towards mental health **are changing**.

2) Past simple

The past simple can be used to narrate a series of events, and so is commonly used in the descriptive sections of reflective writing:

> I **started** my placement in June.
> An elderly patient **was admitted**.

In the first sentence, the agent of the action (I) is important, reflected in the active verb form; in the second sentence, the exact identity of the agent (the person who admitted the patient) is unknown or unimportant in this case, hence the passive verb form.

The past simple is also common when reporting on particular studies or methodologies when reviewing the literature, with the passive voice frequently occurring in the latter, as agency can be presumed:

Graham et al (2015) **found** that side-effects worsened over time.
The subjects **were interviewed** over a period of six months.

3) Present perfect

The present perfect relates an action or a state to the present in some way.

There **has been** a great deal of research in this area.

(This has happened over a time period stretching to the present time.)

The government **has committed** itself to improved funding of the NHS.

(This happened some time before the present moment, but we are not concerned with the precise time – we are more concerned with *what* has happened, not *when*.)

4) Future verb forms

There is no single future verb form in English; many forms are used to refer to the future, depending on how the action is viewed.

This policy **will have** an adverse effect on the recruitment of nurses.

(a prediction)

I**'m meeting** my mentor next week.

(an arrangement)

I**'m going to** contact a Marie Curie nurse to find out more about palliative care for terminal cancer patients.

(an intention)

These verb forms are very common in the concluding sections of reflections, when considering planned actions and future practice.

Further reading

Bottomley, J (2014) *Academic writing for international students of science.* London: Routledge.

Caplan, N (2012) *Grammar choices for graduate and professional writers.* Ann Arbour, MI: University of Michigan Press.

Answer key

Chapter 2, Reflective practice

Critically evaluating reflective frameworks

Task, Comparing and contrasting reflective frameworks (Page 21)

BORTON	GIBBS	JOHNS
What?	Description; feelings	Focus on a description of an experience that seems significant in some way. How was I feeling and what made me feel that way? How do I NOW feel about this experience?
So what?	Evaluation; analysis	Which issues are significant and need attention? How do I interpret the way people were feeling and why they felt that way? What was I trying to achieve and did I respond effectively? What were the consequences of my actions on the patients, others and myself? What factors influenced the way I was/am feeling, thinking and responding to the situation? What knowledge informed me or might have informed me? To what extent did I act for the best and in tune with my values? How does the situation connect with previous experiences?

BORTON	GIBBS	JOHNS
Now what?	Conclusion; action plan	How might I reframe the situation and respond more effectively if a similar situation were to reoccur? What would be the consequences of alternative actions for the patients, others and myself? What factors might constrain me when responding in new ways? Am I more able to support myself and others better as a consequence? What insights have I gained? Am I more able to realise desirable practice?

The language of reflection

Task, Identifying useful words and phrases (Pages 31–33)

1) Reflection on current knowledge and attitudes – E

2) Describing feelings – B

3) Describing reactions to a situation or incident – C

4) Explaining feelings and reactions – A

5) Highlighting important points – F

6) Signalling how the situation or event has challenged previous thinking – G

7) Impact on practice – D

Chapter 4, Critical writing

What does it mean to write critically?

Task, Identifying critical use of language (Page 50)

1) **It seems that** nurses are under **significant** pressure to demonstrate that their work improves outcomes, while at the same time being cost effective. In order to meet **these challenges**, nurses **must** ensure that their practice is research informed.

2) Midwives **may** need to develop additional skills when working in rural and remote areas. This **could** involve skills around the support of teenage mothers and families.

3) **In conclusion**, there have been a number of recent high-profile cases of abuse involving the elderly or those with learning disabilities. While these **almost undoubtedly** involve a minority of practitioners, they **clearly demonstrate** the

need for a renewed commitment to patient care and safety throughout the health and social care professions.

4) The **limited benefits** associated with the use of acupuncture during childbirth **should** be weighed against the cost of providing this treatment.

5) The authors **question** the effectiveness of many of the healthcare programmes that have recently been introduced to target the homeless.

Task, Identifying critical essay writing (Pages 51–56)

1) and 2) see below

This part of the essay title allows you to be descriptive. (Note the word 'outline'.)	**Outline current practices on handwashing in healthcare settings and critically evaluate the extent to which handwashing practices can reduce healthcare-acquired infection.**	This part of the essay title demands that you are critical ('critically evaluate'), thus you cannot be merely descriptive when talking about the impact of handwashing practices on healthcare-acquired infections.

3) and 4) see below

	Introduction	
Words and phrases like 'however', 'although', 'on the other hand', 'despite this', and 'nonetheless' signal that the student knows there is more than one side to an argument or perhaps that the literature is inconsistent	Technological advances have greatly improved the treatment of many diseases and disorders. <u>However</u>, these advances are often undermined by the transmission of infections within healthcare settings, <u>in particular</u>, those resulting from antimicrobial-resistant strains of disease-causing microorganisms, which are now endemic in many healthcare environments (Allegranzi et al, 2011; Loveday et al, 2014). In 2009, healthcare-associated infection (HCAI) affected 5–15 per cent of hospitalised patients in the developed world (WHO, 2009). This figure rises to 9–37 per cent for critically ill patients in intensive care units (ICUs), who are particularly susceptible to HCAI. The most frequently occurring HCAIs affecting these patients are urinary tract infection, surgical site infection, bloodstream infection and pneumonia (WHO, 2009). Studies report higher rates in developing countries, <u>although</u>, according to the World Health Organization, this data, mostly collected in single hospital studies, is a less reliable indicator of wider trends. The huge personal, social and financial costs associated with HCAI have led to a growing public awareness of the threat, and of the need for urgent solutions.	Stating that technological progress does not solve every problem 'in particular' – specifying a particular type of infection Drawing attention to the fact that things are not as simple as they might seem and that evidence must be scrutinised

Drawing on the evidence base, but in a cautious way ('indicates')

{ Epidemiological evidence indicates that hand-transmission is a major contributing factor in the acquisition and spread of HCAI (Loveday et al, 2014). <u>For this reason</u>, healthcare workers' hand hygiene is traditionally considered as the single most important factor in the reduction of HCAI (Gould et al, 2017). Studies on the effects of handwashing protocols in healthcare settings date back to the mid-1800s (WHO, 2009), <u>but</u> it was <u>not until</u> 2001 that the first national evidence-based guidelines for preventing HCAI in NHS hospitals, including hand hygiene as one of its principal interventions, were introduced by the Department of Health in the UK (Loveday et al, 2014).

Providing a rationale for the subsequent claim

Identifying an interesting point, implicitly questioning why this took so long ('but', 'not until')

This essay will begin by outlining current handwashing practices in healthcare settings, with particular reference to national NHS guidelines. It will then examine current evidence, including systematic reviews, in order to critically evaluate the extent to which particular practices can reduce HCAI. The main focus will be on the effectiveness of cleaning agents and the issue of compliance. It will conclude with suggestions on recommendations for nursing practice and suggestions regarding which areas can be usefully investigated further.

Signals the organisation of the argument developed in the essay, clearly linked to the essay question itself

Current guidelines on hand hygiene

Strong claim, backed up by evidence (Sax et al citation)

Globally, one of the most influential frameworks for training, auditing and feedback regarding hand-hygiene practice is the World Healthcare Organization's (WHO) 'Five moments for hand hygiene' (Sax et al, 2007). It has been adopted in many countries, often with local modifications. In the UK, NHS guidelines for preventing HCAIs, developed by a nurse-led team of researchers and specialists, were first introduced in 2001, and updated in 2007 (Loveday et al, 2014). These national guidelines are evidence-based 'broad principles of best practice' which need to be integrated into local contexts (Loveday et al, 2014, p 51). Evidence-based guidelines <u>must</u> be carefully monitored and frequently updated as new evidence and technologies emerge, and Loveday et al, commissioned by the Department of Health, reviewed the existing evidence and found that the 2007 guidelines remained 'robust, relevant and appropriate' <u>on the whole</u> (2014, p 51). <u>However</u>, they did put forward a number of new recommendations,

Strong claim, followed by an example of close monitoring and updating

Analysis of the researchers' response to the existing guidelines

'on the whole': indicates a limitation

as well as proposals for adjustments to existing recommendations.

The standard principles governing the guidelines are based around five distinct interventions (Loveday et al, 2014):

- hospital environment hygiene;
- hand hygiene;
- use of personal protective equipment;
- safe use and disposal of sharps;
- principles of asepsis.

Reminds the reader of the limited scope of the essay {

This essay focuses on the second of these: hand hygiene. The current national guidelines on handwashing, as outlined by Loveday et al (2014), are summarised below.

The guidelines require that healthcare workers:

- decontaminate their hands with soap and water or, in some circumstances, an alcohol-based hand rub (ABHR), at key points such as before and after each episode of patient contact or care;
- wear short sleeves, remove all hand jewellery, keep finger nails short, clean and free from polish or false nails, and cover cuts and abrasions with waterproof dressings;
- employ effective handwashing techniques involving three stages: preparation, washing and rinsing, and drying;
- regularly use an emollient hand cream to offset potential skin irritation from decontamination products;
- have access to alcohol-based hand rub at the point of care;

Identifying the focus of the new recommendations, italics providing emphasis {

- have access to regular training on hand hygiene.

New recommendations by Loveday et al focus on *education and promotion* of the guidelines:

- 'Local programmes of education, social marketing, and auditing and feedback should be refreshed regularly and promoted by senior managers and clinicians to maintain focus, engage staff and produce sustainable levels of compliance'.

(Loveday et al, 2014, p 54).

Drawing attention to an important point (further emphasised by use of italics) {

It is notable that other additions to the guidelines focus on wider *inclusivity*, with requirements that patients and relatives be included in the process:

- Patients and relatives should be provided with information regarding the need for hand hygiene and how to keep their own hands clean.
- Patients should be offered the opportunity to clean their hands at key points such as before meals or after using the toilet, with appropriate products being made available.

Interpretation of the literature, identifying patterns and gaps

The guidelines are evidence based and set out broad principles, but within these, <u>there are still some areas of doubt</u>, <u>in particular</u>, regarding the comparative effectiveness of cleaning agents and the best way to achieve compliance among healthcare workers.

Cleaning agents

The evidence regarding the effectiveness of particular handwashing agents <u>shows no clear pattern</u>. Turner et al (2010) reported that 65 per cent of ethanol hand sanitisers were more effective in removing Rhinovirus that soap and water. <u>However</u>, Grayson et al (2009) and Oughton et al (2009) reported that soap and water was more effective than ABHR for H1N1 influenza virus and *C. difficile*, respectively. Other studies report no significant difference. The review of national guidelines conducted by Loveday et al (2014) found that, overall, there is no compelling evidence to support a particular type of antiseptic handwashing agent, or to suggest that the use of these is preferable to liquid soap. <u>They conclude that</u> it is not possible to establish a causal relationship between ABHR and reductions in HCAIs.

Analysis of the evidence, with some contrasting of disparate points of view

Emphasis

<u>In fact</u>, ABHR is reported to be ineffective in some situations, and <u>even</u> in studies which appear to suggest the superior effectiveness of ABHR, closer investigation often reveals that its use is in fact <u>only</u> one of a number of interventions.

'only' is a small but important word which signals limitations

'even' is a small but important word which signals that what follows may be surprising

Compliance

Loveday et al (2014) <u>stress the importance of</u> compliance in their updated guidelines, <u>but compliance is notoriously difficult to assess</u>: self-reporting <u>can lead to</u> overestimation (Biran et al, 2008), and the presence of an observer <u>can lead to</u> biased results (Pedersen et al, 1986; Ram et al, 2010). <u>It is therefore necessary</u> to treat reported figures on compliance with caution. <u>However</u>, available figures suggest that healthcare workers often comply poorly with handwashing guidelines (Allegranzi and Pitter, 2009). One recent systematic

Cautious use of the evidence

Drawing attention to problems interpreting evidence

review estimated compliance to be between 48 and 72 per cent in high-income countries and between 5 and 25 per cent in low-income countries (Freeman et al, 2014), with an overall mean of <u>only</u> 19 per cent.

'only' is a small but important word which signals limitations

There is <u>some</u> evidence that clear handwashing guidelines and protocols can improve nurses' compliance with hand-hygiene recommendations (Sax et al, 2007; Fox et al, 2015). The systematic implementation of particular guidelines or protocols is known as a *multi-modal approach*. <u>Possibly</u> the most well-known of these is the WHO's 'My five moments for hand hygiene', which, <u>according to</u> Sax et al, 'bridges the gap between scientific evidence and daily health practice and provides a solid basis to understand, teach, monitor and report hand hygiene practices' (Sax et al, 2007, pp 9–10).

Cushioning the claim with caution

Drawing on the evidence base, but 'some' signals caution/ limitations

Drawing on the literature for support

<u>However</u>, according to the most recent Cochrane systematic review on hand hygiene (Gould et al, 2017), the best way to achieve compliance with current recommendations on hand hygiene <u>is yet to be established</u>. Both single-intervention strategies and combinations of strategies, many based on WHO recommendations, have been shown to improve hand-hygiene compliance in many healthcare settings. <u>However</u>, <u>it remains unclear</u> which strategy or combination of strategies is most effective in a particular context (Gould et al, 2017).

Claim, supported by the literature, that the evidence is inconclusive

With the evidence on compliance inconclusive, it's difficult to specify what strategies should be implemented in healthcare settings

Conclusion

In conclusion, clear handwashing guidelines and protocols are provided in many healthcare settings, including the NHS, and these <u>may make a significant contribution towards</u> the prevention of HCAI <u>as part of</u> an overall hygiene strategy <u>if</u> they are strictly implemented, and regularly monitored and updated. <u>The evidence indicates that</u> cleanliness itself is more important than the method of cleaning; <u>much research has been conducted</u> on cleaning agents <u>yet no clear winner has emerged</u>. However, compliance <u>emerges as a key factor</u>, and <u>it seems that</u> clear guidelines and protocols <u>can go some way</u> to improving this, <u>although it remains unclear</u> which particular approaches bring most success. <u>While organisational action is vital</u>, <u>it is also important that</u> nurses and other healthcare workers take personal responsibility and closely follow patient safety aspects of the Code (2015), <u>especially</u> 19: 'Be aware of, and reduce as far as possible, any potential for harm associated with your practice'.

Objective summary statement of the evidence which clearly reflects the uncertainties associated with the topic; note the use of small but important words like 'may', 'if', 'yet', 'seems', 'can'

Critical application to practice

Task Identifying opportunities for criticality (Page 56)

Introduction

- Define long-term conditions. *descriptive*
- Give contextual background particularly relating to long-term conditions in older people (most common = diabetes, chronic obstructive airways disease, hypertension, heart disease, etc). Dementia could be included? *descriptive*
- The focus is on those who care for/support older people with LTCs. Stress that the assignment needs to focus on registered nurses – to do this probably need to discuss other workers who do 'nursing' but are not nurses (healthcare assistants, care workers, support workers, etc). *will involve critical perspective on what nursing is and what nurses are; not all nursing is done by nurses*
- Identify any relevant policy/government documents. *danger of being too descriptive here – should be a critical appraisal, eg what impact they have, how they have been interpreted and applied*
- Explain how you intend to answer the question posed (signpost)

Main section

- Determine what would be deemed to be 'effective' care – suspect things like quality of life and fewer hospital or GP appointments would be good outcomes. *critically determine*
- Likely self-management would play a big role here. (In dementia, may be relatives/carers who do most of self-management.)
- Look for literature on the extent to which registered nurses support self-management. Probably best to look at who supports self-management in general in older people and see if registered nurses feature highly; if not, could argue registered nurses don't make unique contribution. *critical element*
- Outline key things registered nurses can do that other care workers can't (assessments, meds management, possibly even prescribing) when trying to argue for *unique* contribution. *critical element*

Summary/Conclusion

- Bring it all together for the reader, perhaps summarising the previous section in a paragraph. *mostly descriptive*
- Draw a strong conclusion relating to registered nurses' *unique* contribution (or not, as the case may be). *evaluative summary statement*
- Think about implications for future practice/changing future practice. *critical element*

Index